TENNIS
for
Experienced Players

Robert Gensemer
Edinboro University of Pennsylvania

MP

Morton Publishing Company
925 W. Kenyon Avenue, Unit 12
Englewood, Colorado 80110

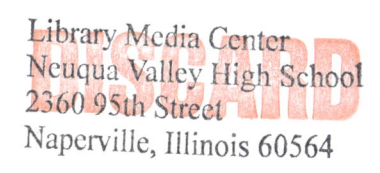

Copyright © 1994 Morton Publishing Company

ISBN: 0-89582-273-3

10 9 8 7 6 5 4 3 2 1

All rights reserved. No part of this publication may be reproduced, stored in a retrieval system, or transmitted, in any form or by any means, electronic, mechanical, photocopying, recording, or otherwise, without the prior written permission of the copyright owner.

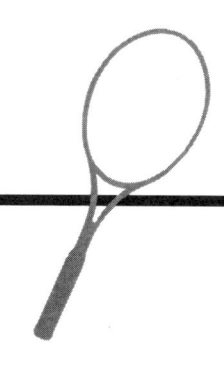

CONTENTS

Preface   vii

Chapter One:
   How To Play Dynamic Tennis   1

Chapter Two:
   Hit Decisive Groundstrokes   11

Chapter Three:
   Spin and Power For the Serve   33

Chapter Four:
   Designed Service Returns   49

Chapter Five:
   Controlling the Forecourt   59

Chapter Six:
   Hitting Point-Winning Lobs   73

Chapter Seven:
   Making Extraordinary Shots Ordinary   83

Chapter Eight:
   Taking Charge of Singles Matches: 93

Chapter Nine:
   Strategic Strength for Doubles   107

Chapter Ten:
   How To Be Mentally Tough   119

Chapter Eleven:
   Realistic Practice   127

Chapter Twelve:
   The Advantage of High-Tech Equipment   135

Appendix A:
   Aerobic Conditioning for Tennis   139

Appendix B:
   A Brief History of the Game   145

Appendix C:
   The National Tennis Rating Program   149

Appendix D:
   A Self-Appraisal Checklist of Skill   51

Appendix E:
   The Rules of Tennis   157

Index   161

ACKNOWLEDGMENTS

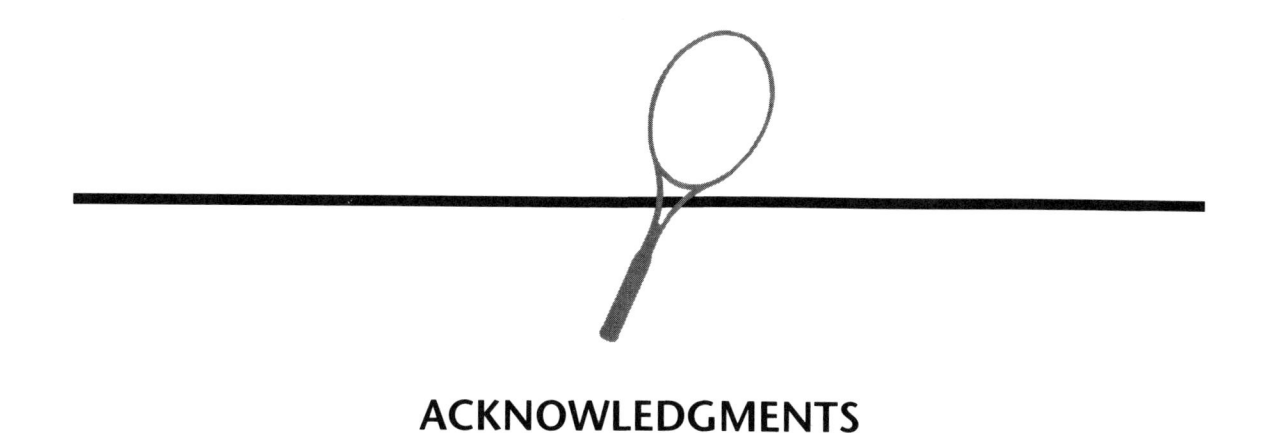

The author extends his gratitude to the many people who gave willingly of their time and talents to assist in this book. Special thanks go to Kelly Erven and Thinnus Verdoes, who are the players in most of the photographs. Darryl Wisnia was the artist for the illustrations.

Preface

This book is for experienced players who want to become better, even excellent! It is for everyone who wants to achieve the satisfaction of a skill well done.

You have had your apprenticeship. Your blisters have turned to calluses, and you play often enough to wear out a couple pair of shoes a year. You can prolong a rally, hit with intent to an opponent's weaker side, angle sharply hit cross-court shots, and your serve has convincing pace with reasonable accuracy. You are ready to become a complete player.

This book will help. It will guide you to the next level of play with no-nonsense descriptions of techniques for skillful execution. It is based throughout on sound principles of physics, coupled with disclosures of the styles of the best players in the game, and tempered to be applicable to all developing players. The writings are not excessively detailed, but there is completeness in the formulas that will make you an expressive, dynamic, effective player.

There is also full attention to the strategies of play, so there is never any doubt about where to hit the ball, or what kind of shot to hit, or where to be. And there is counsel for your brain, telling of how to develop a mental readiness to gather all your resources for a competitive flair.

In all, this book is intended to help you become a better, more perceptive, more self-appraising player. It is not a substitute for practice, but rather a compliment to it. These pages contain useful information. So do books on brain surgery. But neither is enough, without practice and guided instruction, to assure a successful performance.

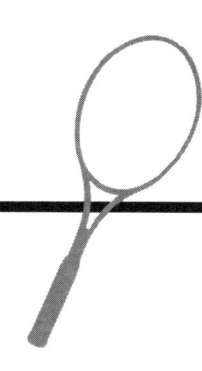

Chapter One

How To Play Dynamic Tennis

We all want to be good at tennis.

No, we want to be **excellent**!

But accomplished playing ability does not just happen. It evolves. Time and practice are the requisites. The foundation is in the mechanics of motion, tempered by that fine human quality of being able to give compelling rhythm and electricity to the movements of tennis.

It all begins inside our heads. Splendid tennis requires the right **attitude** — of open-mindedness, of willingness to experiment, of readiness to hit with flair, and even some recklessness. Cultivated play will not evolve from a conservative approach of push-the-ball-over-the-net. Instead, the mental component must be **permissive**, giving full sanction to the body to experience new techniques, to profit from mistakes, and to be unconstrained.

There is also a **physical** feeling. To become flamboyant at tennis, one cannot play with machine-like insensitivity. It simply isn't that kind of a game. It's actually possible to be relatively "perfect" in form, and yet have inert results. Rather, it's imperative to get caught up in the **flow** of the game, thus to be a free hitter and play with spontaneous enthusiasm.

To be a crafty tennis player, you must become alert to the biofeedback of your own nervous system. You must become sensitive to your own inner self — to literally get inside your muscles, to monitor their activity, and more effectively control their movements. As a result, you'll perceive the racket as part of you, and the ball will jump off the strings with a new liveliness. Best of all, you will have opened your mind and body for spirited play and genuinely personified refinements of talent.

Watch accomplished players. They have certain traits in common.

- Better players **look** different — they appear more relaxed, yet alive and energetic.
- They are **poised**, in full command of their physical responses.
- They are confident and self-assured. They believe that they can play well. They think **positively**, not negatively, about their game.
- The racket seems to be a part of them — a literal extension of their hitting arm.
- Every stroke is **fluid** — not segmented into parts, but rather a continuous, rhythmical, flowing motion.
- They hit the ball with their **entire body**, not just with their arm.
- Their style is often free-lanced, not incessantly bound by a compulsion to always have perfect, picturebook form.
- They focus their attention on the **ball**, without agonizing over their opponent, or the net, or the baseline, or a previous errant shot.
- They **enjoy** the game and want to be challenged. They relish every chance to hit the ball.
- They are mentally, as well as physically, stimulated by the game.

Excellent tennis requires an agreeable harmony of physical aptitude and mental readiness. But sometimes we get impatient, wanting all our tennis weapons to fall into quick mastery. So we need to remind ourselves of some basics, particularly if it's early in the season, which support the advanced skills we seek. Following are some factors which need constant reminder of mind and muscle.

STAY RELAXED

Tense muscles produce rigid shots — nervous shots that are scattered and faulty. The first requisite for smooth, coordinated hitting is to remain relaxed — not lethargic, but calm.

Consciously untie your muscles. Go limber — not to where you're unresponsive, but relaxed and ready. Stay loose, yet alive and energetic. Keep that feeling no matter what kind of shot you are about to hit. Slacken your body; it will help you not only to hit more imaginative shots, but also to enjoy the game more.

THINK RHYTHM AND TIMING

Generate a sense of rhythm and timing. Tennis isn't weight lifting — it's more like a dance. Create an image in your mind of gliding through your strokes, then hit with spontaneous flowing. Give each swing a fluid motion with an unhurried start, a solid middle, and an unrestrained finish — especially the finish. You'll get greater depth and accuracy when you complete your stroke with a follow-through that lets the head of the racket continue into the direction of the shot.

Relaxation, rhythm, and timing. They will **allow** you to hit more dynamic serves, more decisive groundstrokes, and more freewheeling overheads.

BE READY TO RESPOND

Maintain a ready-to-react attitude with a low center of gravity. Use the same cat-like, poised-to-pounce position you would when guarding an opponent in basketball, or playing shortstop in softball. Keep your racket forward, elbows held in front of your hips. Relax your shoulders, and ease your grip on the racket.

Try adding "bounce" to your readiness. Instead of keeping your weight at rest between shots, energize it by bouncing rhythmically on your toes. Feel the alertness go from your toes up through your legs and hips, all the way into your shoulders. Use your thighs to give you the life, like you did when speed-skipping a rope. It will give your whole body more voltage and your reactions more quickness. Just be careful not to get caught airborne when your opponent is hitting the ball.

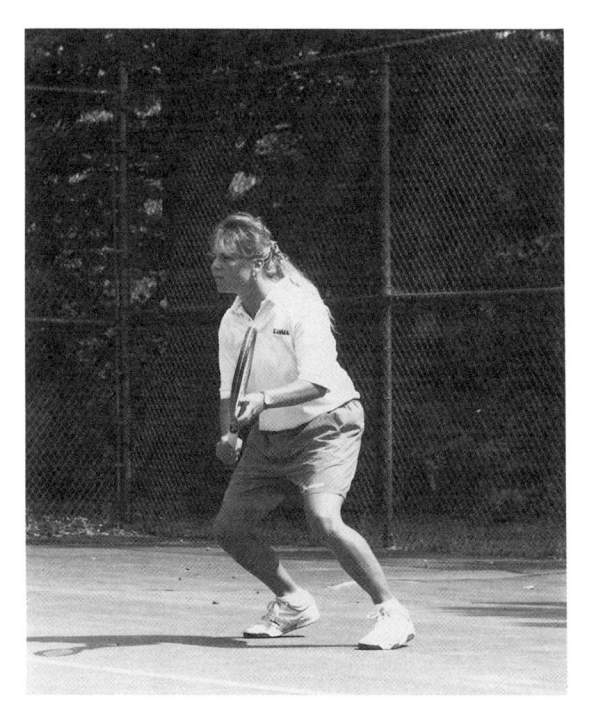

Here's a player in the middle of a rally. There's plenty of life and spring-like energy in this ready-to-respond position.

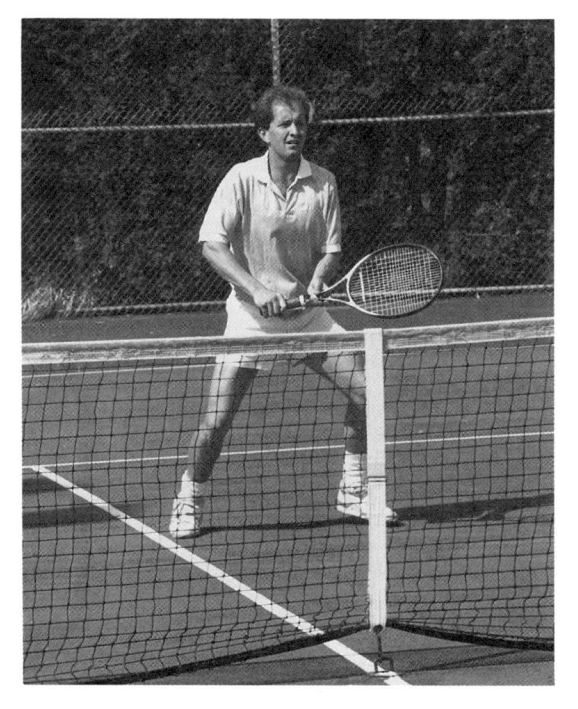

*Keep this alert attitude of being ready to spring into a response. Stay animated to **move** — to pivot, or accelerate, or change directions.*

COIL AND UNCOIL

If there is a single dimension which underlies effective play in tennis, it is the fluid, continuous motion through a windup for the backswing and an unwinding into the foreswing. The body **coils** in preparation for the hit, then **uncoils** with rhythm and power. Coil and uncoil. Everything back together — then forward together. It's a compact maneuver for a volley, more sweeping for a groundstroke, freely expressive for a serve. No matter how intense the swing, the movement should be flowing — effortless energy in motion. It makes you a human being, not a machine. It makes tennis a game, not work. And it makes the game a pleasure, not a stressor.

Turn shoulders, arms, hips, racket, all together in a neat, packaged backswing that coils the body ready for uncoiling into the foreswing. This is especially critical for a backhand, where the shoulders play a more important power role.

This whole-body pivot should precede every stroke, including the serve. Relatedly, if you need to chase down a ball hit to the side of the court, the upper body should first rotate to "pull" you into the direction of your run. And, when you're at the net and your opponent crashes a shot directly at you, a quick pivot of the shoulders will help you get away from the onrushing missile and give your arm enough freedom to operate for a retaliatory smack of the ball.

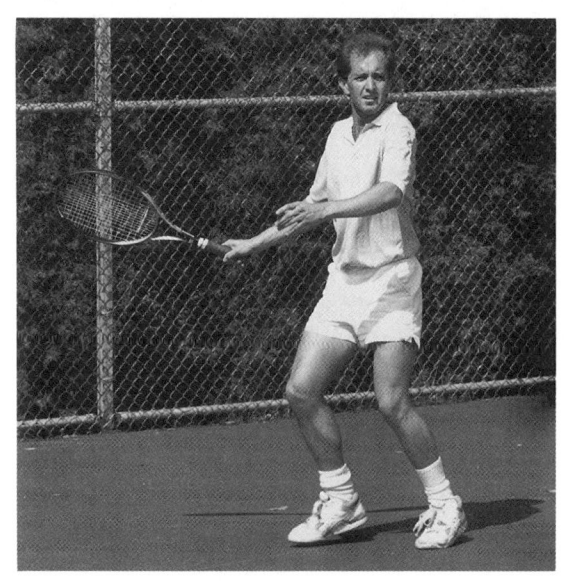

The whole body coiling precedes every stroke. It's a unit turn of shoulders, hips, arms, all together.

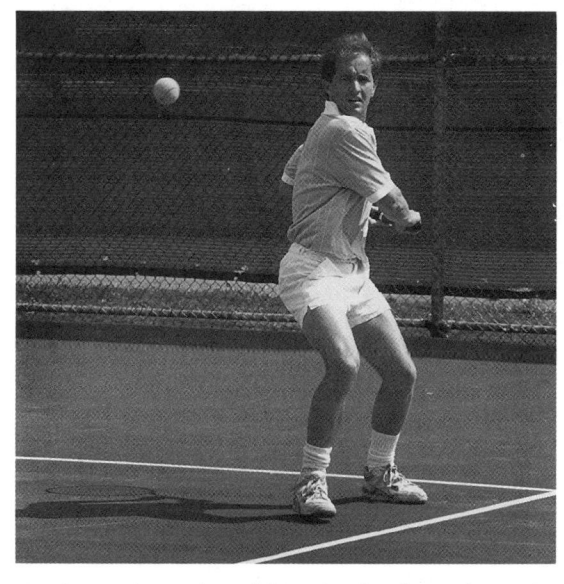

Begin each stroke with a backswing where the whole body pivots, whether it be a coil for a groundstroke . . .

. . . or preparation for a volley . . .

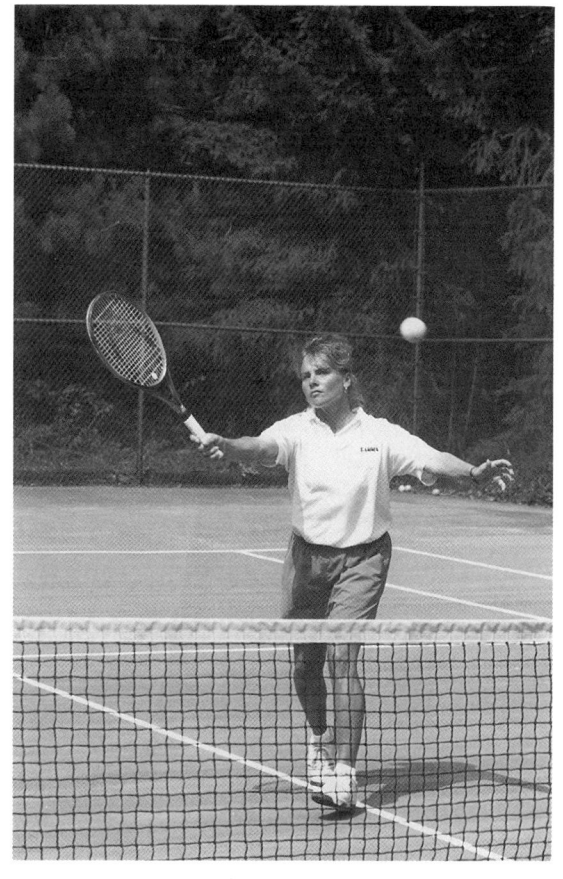

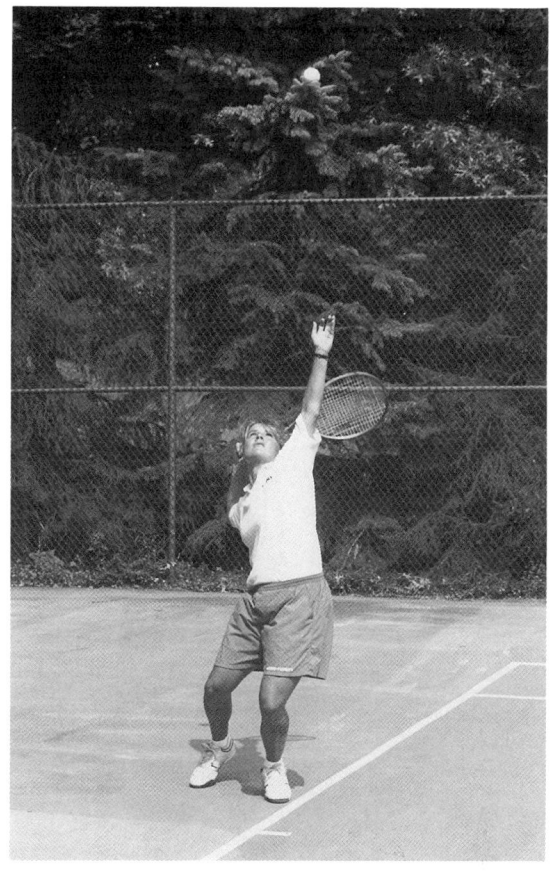

. . . or the windup for a serve.

GO FORWARD AT IMPACT

Whenever there is enough time to collect yourself into effective hitting postion, have your weight going forward — toward the direction of the intended shot — as you contact the ball. Bring everything — racket, arm, shoulders, hips, knees — toward the target as you uncoil into the swing. Reach out and **forward** with the stroke. Feel the energy of your entire body driving toward the spot you want the ball to go.

Even when you must chase down a ball on the run, try to get into position to make your last step directly toward your target. This forward-at-contact impulse is important not only for groundstrokes, but also for serves, overheads, volleys, everything. When you put your entire self into your swing, you will produce a more affirmative shot, and the ball will feel heavier on the strings of your opponent's racket.

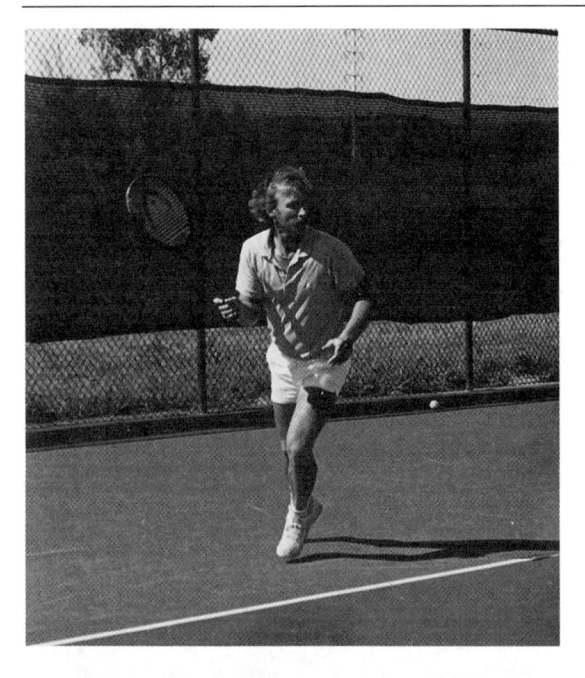

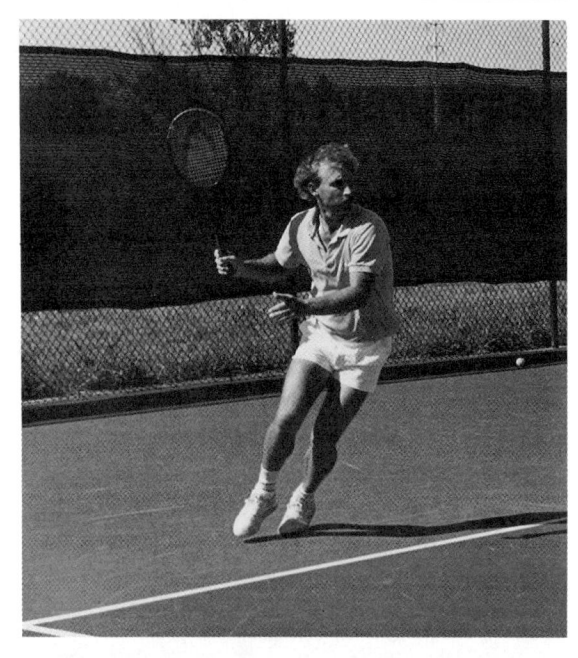

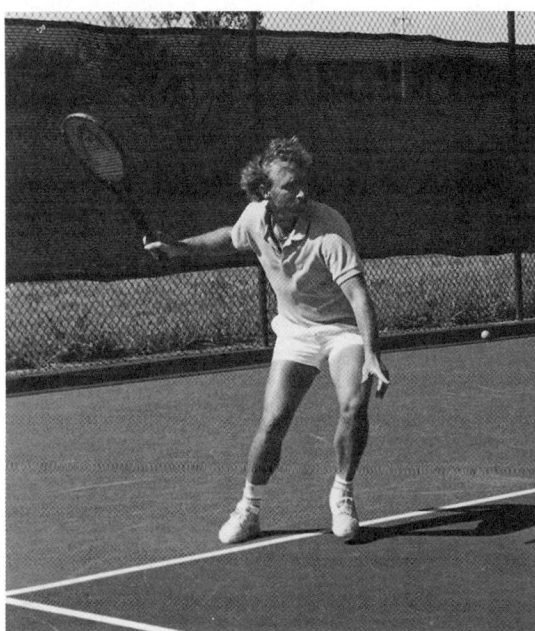

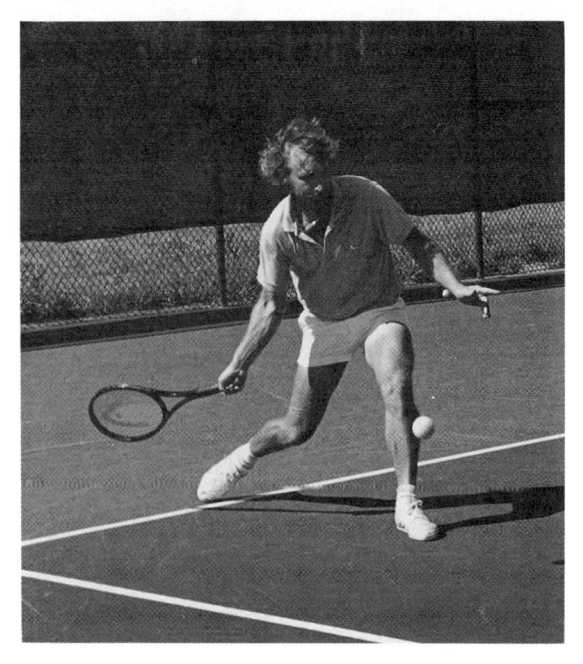

Even when on the move to chase down a ball hit to the side of the court, try to circle your approach so that you can swing your momentum around into the ball while moving forward at impact.

HIT THROUGH THE BALL

It's one of the most commonly used phrases in sports: "hit through the ball." It means, for tennis, to make sure the racket is not quitting its forward speed as it meets the ball. If it does, the ball is unresponsive and lifeless and feels like a rock on the strings. Off-centers hits may twist the racket in your hand, and to compensate you might tighten your grip, thinking you have weak wrists, and your swing will become too stiff.

To give direction to the ball, feel like you're carrying the ball on the strings for as long as possible. Hit forward and **through** the ball. Keep your racket active in the hitting zone — do not let it slow down by holding back on your swing. Allow it to come to a gradual rest only after you complete a solid, flowing hit.

Check your follow-through on groundstrokes. Hold your finish position for a second to see where the racket head is at the end of the swing. It should have come freely around your hitting shoulder.

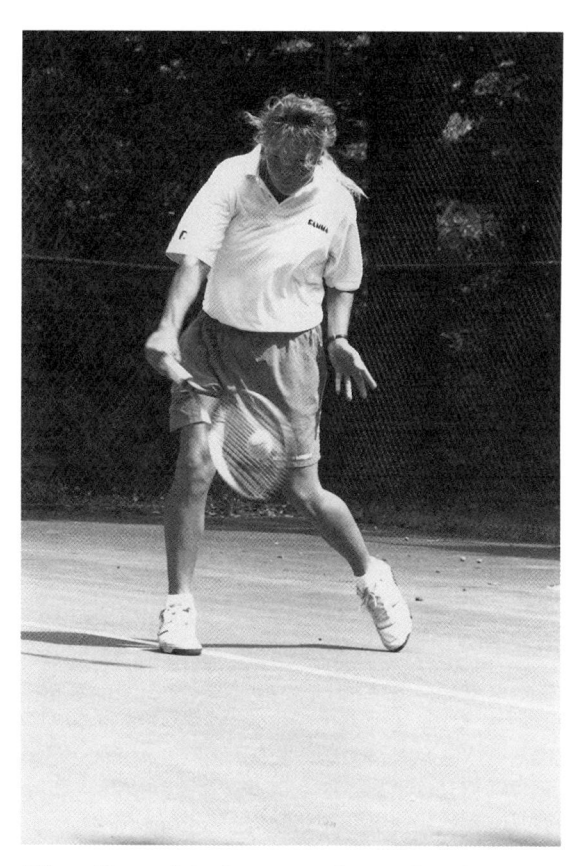

When the weight has gone forward at impact it finishes on the front foot, with the racket completing an unrestricted follow-through.

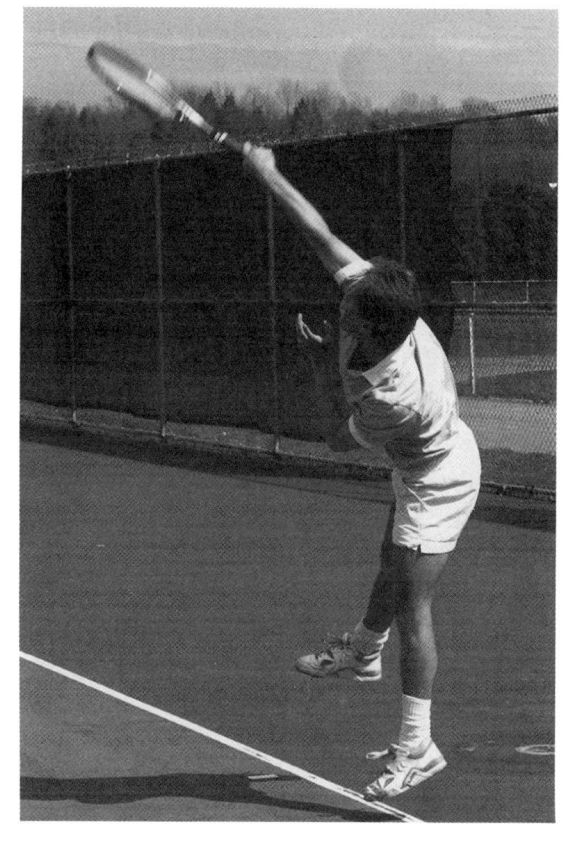

The objective of hitting through the ball with an active racket applies to all strokes, including the serve.

On serves, your follow-through must also be unconstrained, with the racket head finishing down toward the court, indicating that you swung freely at the ball instead of pushing it passively.

On a volley, a lazy racket is a disaster. The ball will overpower the racket, and the stroke will be punchless.

On overheads, if the racket is not lively at contact your shoulder may hunch up and there is hesitancy in the swing. The racket quits — and the ball is listless.

Even on a lob, when you need to lift a soft shot, the racket must come up actively into and through the ball, with the head following the lifted flight of the ball.

BEND YOUR KNEES; KEEP YOUR EYE ON THE BALL

They are the two most timeworn admonitions in tennis.

(1) "Bend your knees." It's difficult to play dynamic tennis when hitting with stilted legs. Planting a stiff forward knee on a groundstroke will jar the whole body and deny a proper weight transfer. Flexed knees (especially the forward leg) will allow a smooth shift of weight toward the target and will allow for a uniform, rhythmical swing. You'll rotate around your front knee instead of having to climb up over it.

Never lock your knees. Not when hitting; not when waiting to hit; not when serving; not when receiving the serve; not at the net. Stiff knees make for stiff shots and an unresponsive body.

(2) "Keep your eye on the ball." You do not really need to see the actual contact of the ball on the racket, but you **do** need to fix your attention on the approaching ball to visually track it into the hitting zone. Focus on the ball as it leaves your opponent's racket, then refocus again after the bounce. Notice how much the ball seems to slow down from its bounce, giving you time to clearly set your sights and organize the coordination of your swing.

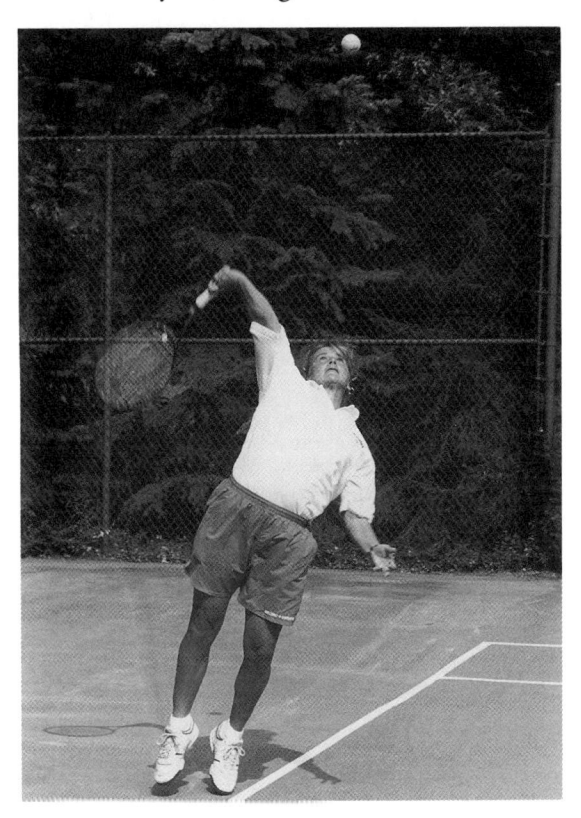

It's especially vital to keep your eye on the ball during the serve, not only watching it hang in the air waiting for you to crash into it, but also seeing the actual impact and the empty space AFTER the hit. Keep your chin up through contact. Say to yourself, "See space!" — and you will almost be able to watch the air come in to fill the space where the ball was before you hit it. That way you'll not drag down your hitting shoulder and lose power.

REMINDERS

1. Relax. Stay limber, yet alert and responsive.
2. Stay lively on your toes. Between exchanges in a rally, stay active with a ready-to-respond attitude.
3. To prepare for any stroke, pivot the whole body as a unit. Coil and uncoil; back together — forward together.
4. Get the whole body into the swing — racket, shoulders, fanny — all moving on-line toward the target at impact.
5. Keep the racket active through the hitting zone. Hit every ball with conviction.
6. Give rhythm to every hit. Produce smooth strokes. Flow through every swing.
7. Let your swing be dynamic, spontaneous, expressive.

PROBLEM SOLVING

Problem	Probable Cause	Solution
Sluggish responses	Tense, static, unready between shots	Be an athlete, prepared in a ready-to-**move** attitude
Tight, jerky shots	Body too stiff	Relax grip; slacken body
	Tense swing or overhitting	Think rhythm and timing during swing
Improper weight transfer	Stiff front leg	Keep legs springy; bend and flex between points
	Not going forward at ball contact	Drive whole body toward target during foreswing
Lifeless shots	Racket quitting in hitting zone	Accelerate the racket into and through the ball. Exaggerate the follow-through
No power	Arm-only swing	Coil and uncoil with whole body; put everything into swing

ON THE COURT

Next time out on the court, give attention to the sensation of rhythm and timing in your swing, emphasizing coiling and uncoiling. Hit convincingly through the ball. During practice hitting, it's easy to be careless — not paying much mind to the design of your strokes. So the ball might get casually struck, perhaps at poor contact points, or with inadequate weight transfer, or with stiff knees, whatever. The hazard is that some ineffective habits, not being of much consequence during a practice knockabout, might filter into becoming part of your regular routine. Every time you hit a ball, your body remembers, to some degree, the swing that it took. Make it remember your **best** style.

Emphasize footwork. Try the "bounce step," where you **unweight** just as your practice partner is about to hit the ball. Take a hopscotch skip-step into a ready-to-respond position, timing it so that you have split your feet and taken weight off your heels just as the ball is being struck. Try it not only for groundstrokes, but also at the net. You'll be less likely to get stuck in a frozen position on any ball, especially when receiving the serve.

Alert your muscles to keep the racket alive, actively moving through the hitting zone — on **all** shots. Help yourself into this habit by going forward at impact. Stay a little further back for a practice rally so you must consciously move up and into each ball, with your whole body giving leverage into the shot.

In particular, use the practice session to give rhythm and timing to every stroke. Make it form and function together. Think of the **art** of tennis. Try to "look good" as you hit. Talk yourself into it. Say "smooooth" as you bring your racket into and through the ball. **float** through your strokes. Then when it feels right, think of **why** it feels right. Let the sensation linger in your muscles, and grant them the freedom to have the same swing for the next ball. Soon, when it's right, you'll **know** it's right.

Chapter Two

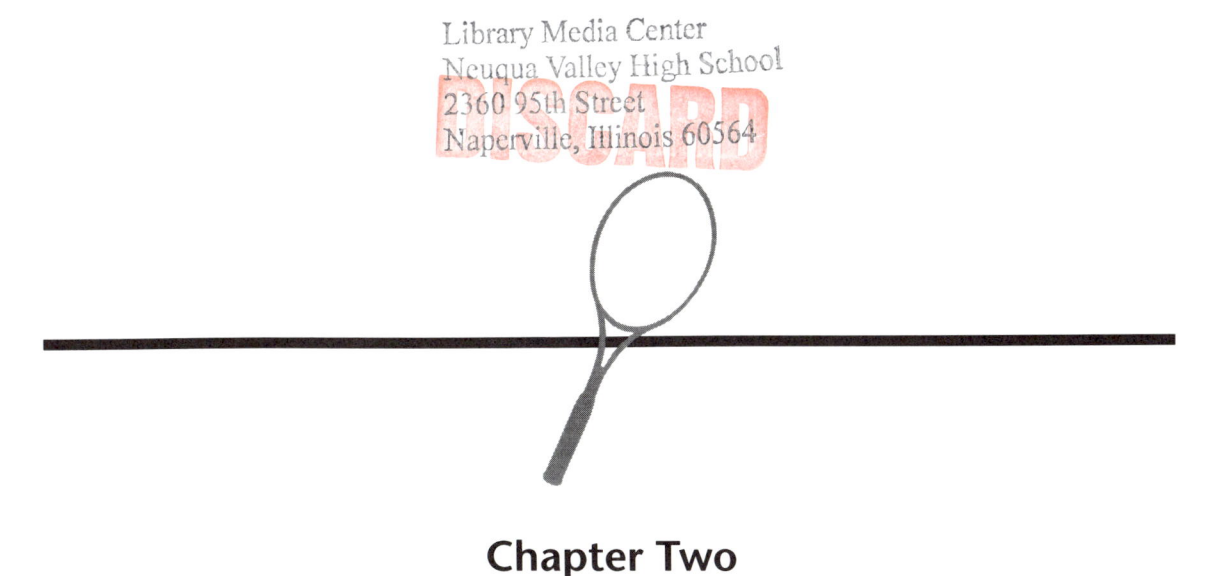

Hit Decisive Groundstrokes

Crush the ball!!

Hit it with infinite authority. Pulverize the ball with convincing swings. Hit it decisively into this corner, then into that corner. Send the ball into submission. Make it behave like a guided missile.

Powerful groundstrokes — shots hit with compelling force — without loss of control; that's a major ingredient for tennis excellence. And happily, power and control are not mutually exclusive.

The best combination, actually, is to generate as much pace as possible without losing any (1) consistency, (2) depth, or (3) placement of the shots. So the strategy is to increasingly add power to one's game until the other dimensions of play begin to break down. Accordingly, if you can hit the ball consistently in the court, keep it deep, and place it where you want to, then you should be adding more pace and spin to your groundstrokes.

EASE THE GRIP

A first requisite for power is to hold the racket loosely. You'll automatically squeeze the racket harder as it approaches the ball. What you do **not** want is to start the swing with an arm-restricting, hammerlock grip. If you lock your wrist, you will reduce the neurological feel of the racket in your hand. The moral, therefore, is: "Loose grip to start — firm grip at contact."

Between points, consciously open your fingers to take any stress out of your hand. And between shots of a continuous rally, keep your grip loose, unbound. Cradle the racket in your opposite hand to take some of its weight out of your hitting arm. During practice, say to yourself, "Loose to start — firm to hit." Eventually you'll develop so much feel for the racket that you'll think you have strings between your fingers.

ACCELERATE THE RACKET

Remember to "hit through the ball." Do it by increasing the velocity of your swing into contact. A racket head that is accelerating at impact will impart more force to the ball than if the racket has the same forward speed, but no acceleration.

Take a positive, determined swing — a good coil and uncoil — and stay tenaciously active through the hitting zone. Make the racket gather momentum so that it comes into the ball while still gaining speed.

You can tell if you're accelerating the racket by how the ball feels on the strings. If the racket is not gaining speed at contact, the ball will feel heavy, like a rock. Off-center hits produce a "twang" — your hand vibrates, and the racket may twist in your grasp. By contrast, with an accelerating racket, the ball will feel like it has virtually no weight. Your feedback will tell you that the racket head has overpowered the moving mass of the ball, rather than vice-versa, and the ball will spring into noticeably livelier flight. It even **sounds** different — a higher pitched "thwack" instead of the dull "thud" that comes from a lazy racket head.

SOURCES OF POWER

How can you get the racket into optimal acceleration, and thus to produce more power? In two ways:

1. **Linear momentum**, resulting from the transfer of weight from the back to the front foot, or at least an active pressing of the body's impulse into the direction of the shot.
2. **Rotary momentum**, coming from the unwinding rotation of the body during the forward swing.

Both work together in a sequential chain of events which, when coordinated correctly, has the following order:

1. With the completion of the windup, the weight pushes off the back foot to begin a forward transfer.
2. Hips move forward and begin to rotate, opening up toward the target.
3. Trunk picks up the rotation.
4. Shoulders rotate.
5. Arm and racket come forward, accelerating into the ball.

The end product of these integrated forces is more than the sum of the parts. But to maximize their effect, they must be performed **sequentially**. Optimal power will not be generated if, for example, the forward swing does not start with a weight transfer. If

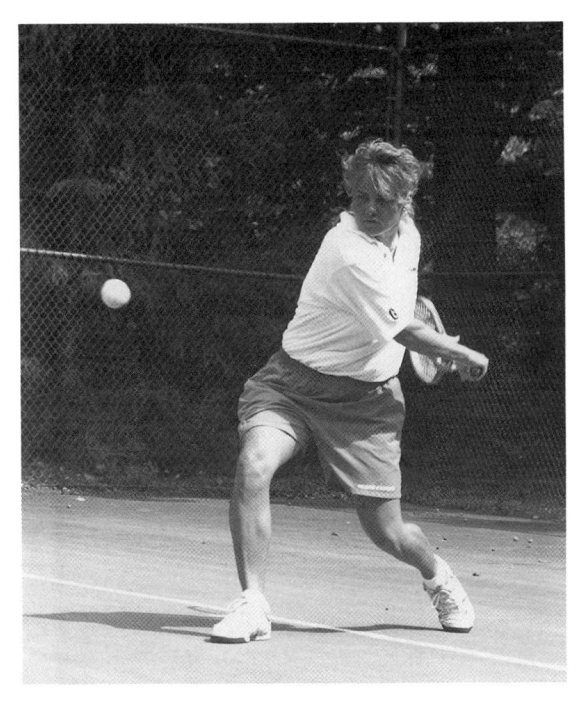

Linear momentum originates from a forward stride and transfer of weight, while . . .

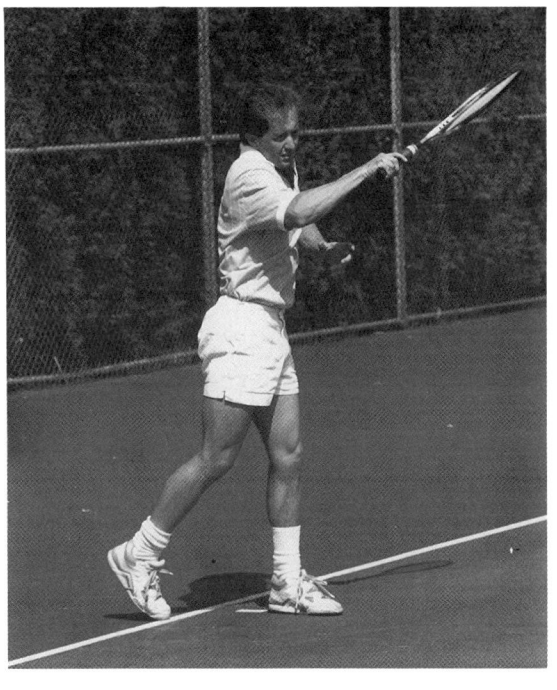

. . . rotary momentum results from an unwinding of the entire body during the forward swing.

the weight stays on the back foot, linear momentum is minimized, and the hitter will be left with only the rotary component to deliver the power. Thus it should be: (1) step, then (2) swing. Linear momentum is derived mostly from the legs, while rotary momentum is a product of the sequential uncoiling of the body.

OPEN UP FOR THE HIT

For rotary momentum to gather its optimal force, the body literally needs to get out of the way of its own hitting arm. Often we are taught to hit forehands out of a closed stance. But when power is an objective, this closed stance will restrict a free-flowing motion since the forward side of the body is now in the way of the follow-through. It also impedes the rotation of the hips; thus racket acceleration at contact is less likely.

Observe the professional players. Given enough time to collect themselves for a forehand, they will generally hit from a variably **open** position. The reason is, in part, to allow the hips and shoulders to add unrestricted rotary momentum to the swing.

So there's a medium somewhere. For a forehand, the body should be opened enough to permit freedom for rotary momentum in the swing, but not so open as to hinder the forward transfer of weight.

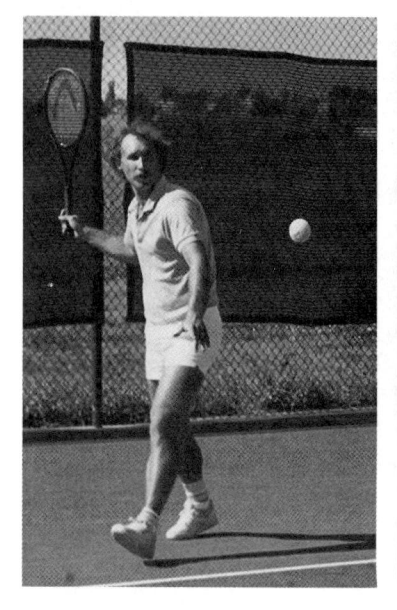

For a forehand, the concept of "stepping into the ball" can be misinterpreted to mean . . .

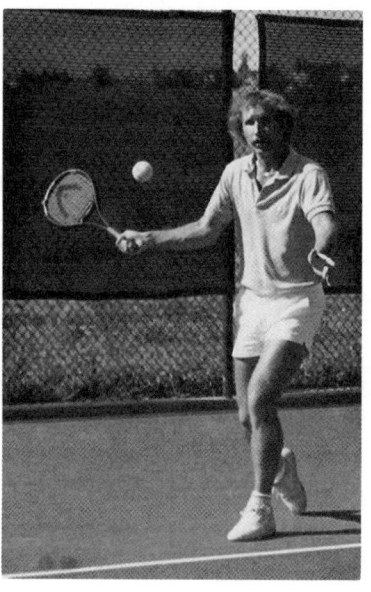

. . . stepping AT the ball, resulting in too much of a closed position that hinders weight transfer ...

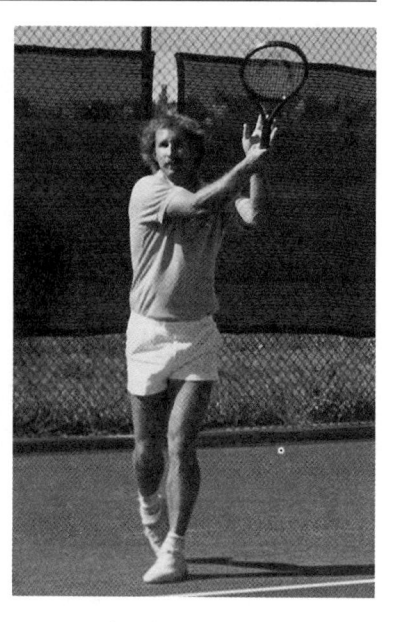

. . . and reduces the free flow of the swing and follow-through.

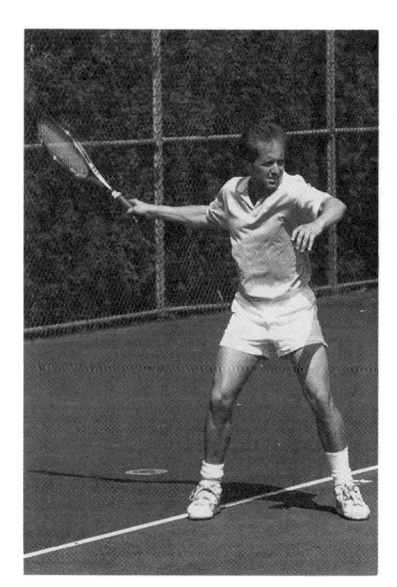

In contrast, when the stride into a forehand provides an open hitting position . . .

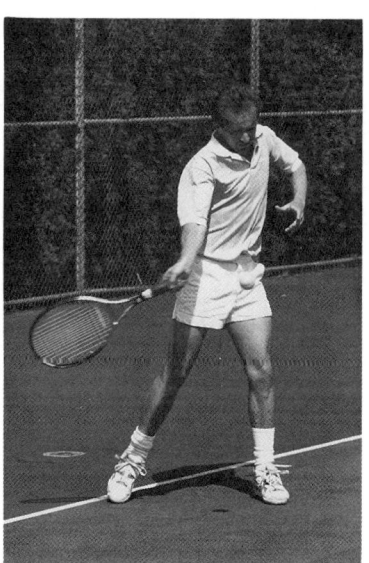

. . . linear momentum is greater, and the unrestricted rotation of the hips allows for . .

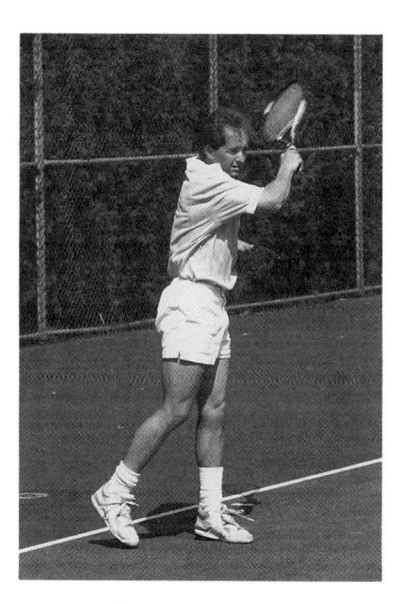

. . . a free swing of sequential body levers to maximize rotary momentum.

For a backhand, an open hitting position is not vital because the swing moves out and away from the body. In fact, an open stance will actually tend to restrict the **backswing** for a backhand. Consequently, a somewhat closed hitting position is more economical for a clean swat at the ball.

Two-handed backhands allow for more versatility in hitting position. With the added impulse of the second arm, rotary momentum is more readily generated irrespective of the body position during the forward swing. Consequently, two-fisted hitters are not as likely to be restricted by a compressed backswing that would otherwise result from an open hitting position.

In theory, two-handed backhands should deliver more force from the cumulative effect of both arms. Since the trunk and the arms pivot as more of a single unit, rotary momentum is increased with less need for strength in the swing. Two arms reinforce each other to give extra leverage to the mechanics of the stroke (see series of photos on next page). But one-handed or two, the driving force of a backhand comes more from the rotary momentum of the shoulders than for a forehand.

THE FLATTENED-ARC SWING

Think of paddling a canoe. To get maximum pull, you take as long a stroke as possible and keep the paddle flat against the direction of the pull. It's the same for a

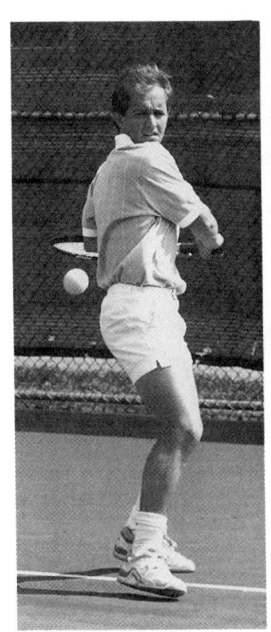

For a backhand, more rotary momentum is needed from the shoulders, thus . . .

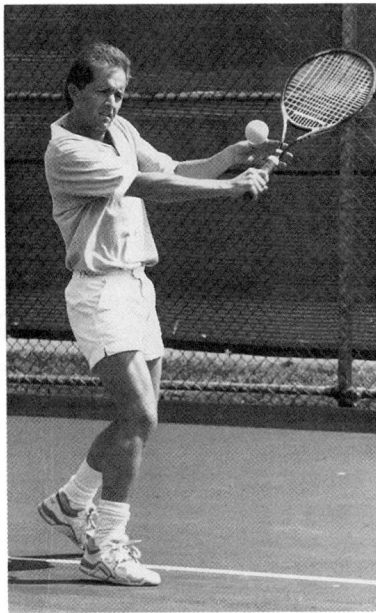

. . . a relatively closed hitting position permits a longer backswing without . . .

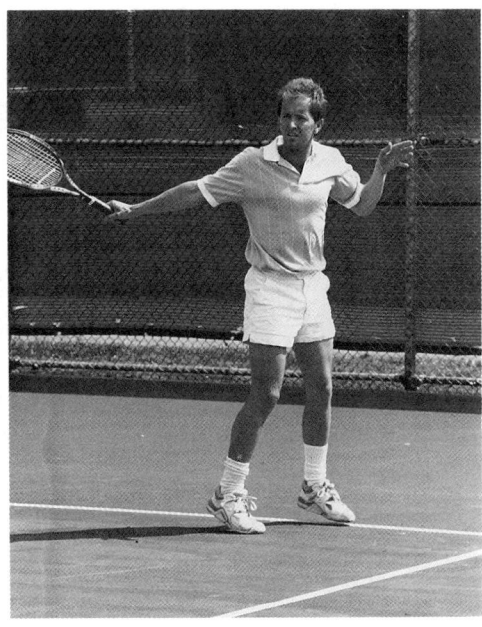

. . . restricting either linear or rotary momentum during the forward swing into the ball.

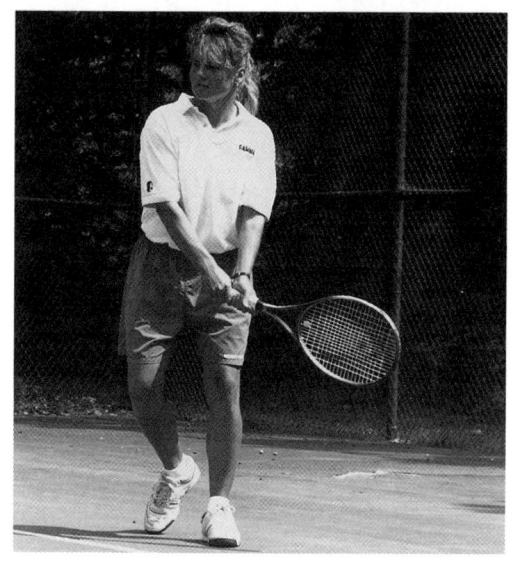

A principle advantage of the two-handed backhand is the power it can generate . . .

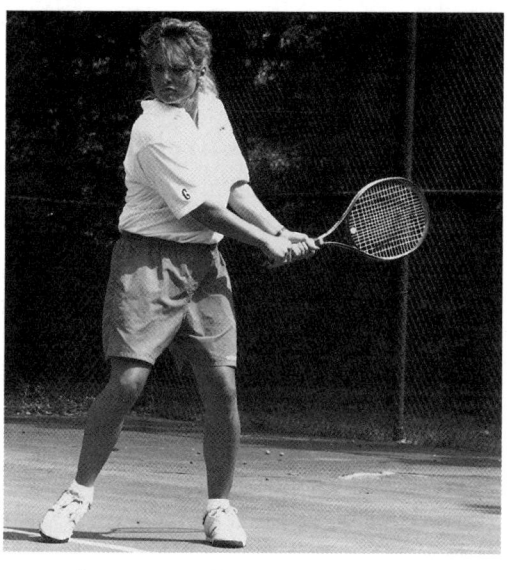

. . . by more effectively transferring the rotary momentum of the trunk and shoulders to the racket.

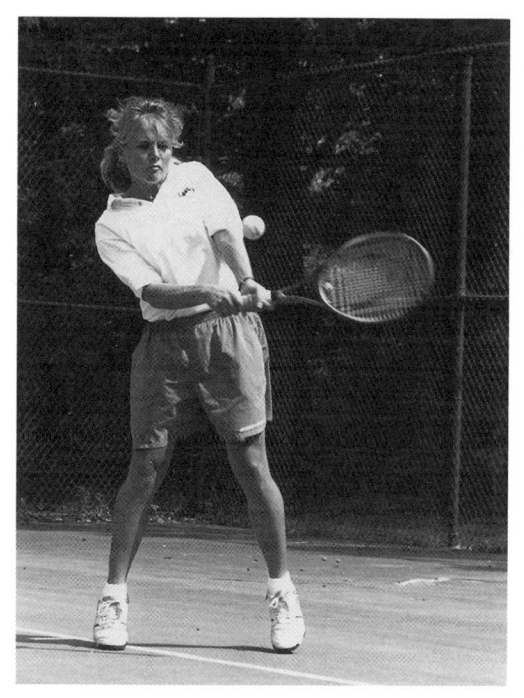

But it still needs linear momentum through a weight transfer to meet the ball out in front . . .

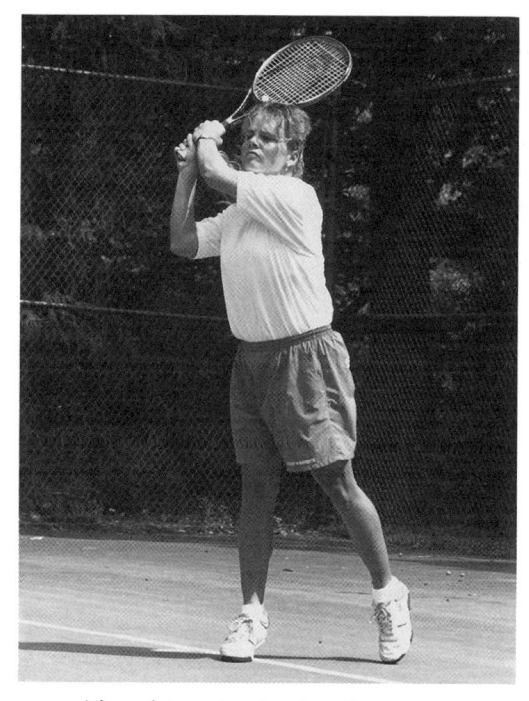

. . . with a determined swing that accelerates the racket into an unrestrained high finish.

NOT THIS   BUT THIS

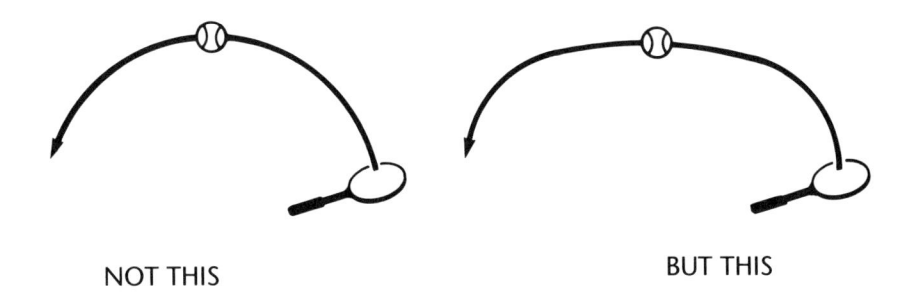

Linear momentum can be increased through a flattened-arc swing as illustrated on the right, compared to a static-arm swing which results in the circular path shown on the left.

groundstroke. To increase effective length and optimize power, the swing should flatten out and lengthen as it approaches the ball, racket face staying square-on to the target.

The racket starts from close in, then moves out and forward through the hitting zone. It begins with the elbow flexed, about the same as it is when held in readiness between points. The arm then **extends**, elbow unbending into the hitting zone. It is a natural, centrifugal response of the arm, and its effect is to lengthen the radius of the swing, thus adding whip to the stroke and power to the ball. As a bonus to this flattened-arc swing the ball can be hit more accurately, since the racket head stays on course toward the target for a longer path through the hitting zone.

GROUNDSTROKE REMINDERS

1. Keep the grip loose to start, firm to hit.
2. Get a good unit turn of the upper body into the windup, especially for backhands.
3. When coiling for a backhand, look over the forward shoulder to sight the approaching ball. Pretend that an arrow extended through both shoulders would point at the ball.
4. Keep your head steady, eyes riveted on the ball into the hitting zone.
5. Unweight your front foot as you coil into the backswing in preparation for forward linear momentum.
6. Keep the swing continuous, with no interruption of the kinetic energy that is building during the windup.
7. Get all your weight into the shot. Accelerate the racket. Explode into the ball.
8. On two-handed backhands, give extra freedom to the rotary momentum of the shoulders.
9. Extend fully through the ball. Bring the racket head toward the target through a flattened-arc swing.
10. Imagine carrying the ball on the strings as long as you can. Think that each ball has three others behind it. Try to thread the racket through all four as you swing.

PROBLEM SOLVING

Problem	Probable Cause	Solution
Erratic shots	Not watching ball	Keep head steady, following ball into hitting zone
Ball feels dead on racket	No acceleration	Drive racket emphatically into ball; do not be tentative
Poor balance	Not getting into effective hitting position	Take small shuffle steps when nearing ball
	Weight held back during contact	Make last step toward the target
Slashing, wraparound swing	Hitting position too closed, especially in forehand	Open the forward stride; press weight toward target
	No linear momentum	Swing through a flattened arc
Minimal linear momentum	No weight shift	Drive entire body toward target during foreswing
	Not generating kinetic force	Press weight toward target first, then release swing
Minimal rotary momentum	Hips restricted from complete turn	Hit from open stance on forehands, only slightly closed on backhands
	Static, one-piece foreswing	Sequentially unwind hips, trunk, shoulders during foreswing

THE ADVANTAGE OF ADDING SPIN

When you can intentionally spin the ball from your groundstrokes, you automatically move up one level in tennis. The most advantageous action is when the ball can be hit with topspin, where the rotation of the ball will send it curving downward toward the court. With topspin you can clear the net with a greater margin of safety, or rip a crushing cross-court forehand that will dip dramatically into the court out of reach of your helpless opponent.

The opposite is backspin, which allows you to drop a soft shot just over the net and have it "sit down" in front of your scrambling rival. Or you can send a backspinning ball to a corner and watch the low hop force your opponent to hesitate in the swing.

Topspin grants the freedom to hit with extra pace and with confidence that the ball will arc into the court no matter how emphatically it is struck. Backspin can be used for touch shots and to take the sting out of opponents' strong shots.

Spin makes your game more versatile, more opportunistic. It allows you to be offensive when the moments are right, and defensive when necessary. All the while, you'll have more influence on the pace of a match and more control over the outcome.

THE EFFECTS OF SPIN

The influencing factor which causes a ball to curve in flight is not what the air does to the ball, but what the ball does to the air. As it spins, the ball grabs a layer of surrounding air molecules and spins them around with it. In flight, this has the effect of changing air pressure around the surface of the ball. If the ball has topspin (where the top surface of the ball is spinning into the direction of its flight), it will be pulling air up over its top surface. As the ball moves forward, this air is flung into a headlong crash with the stationary

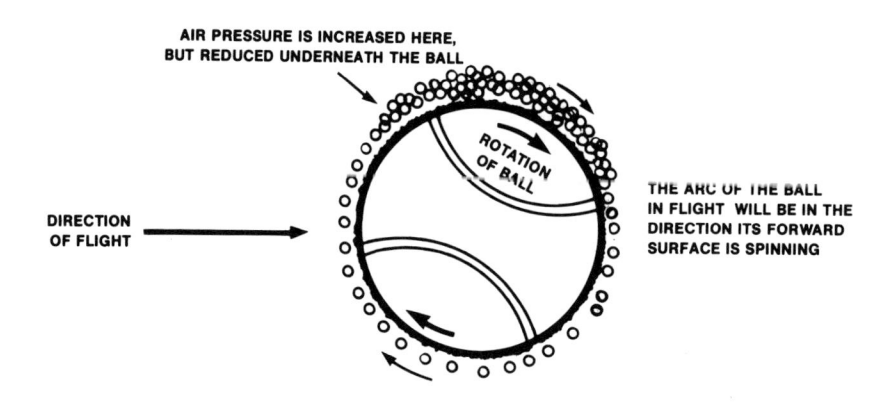

Effects of ball rotation on resulting flight.

atmospheric air. This friction creates a crowding of air molecules on the upper surface of the ball, thereby increasing pressure.

But underneath the ball, the effect is the opposite. The rotating ball is, in flight, pushing air molecules out of the way much in the fashion that a car tire, when accelerating on a dirt road, will kick gravel out behind it. Consequently, there is less crowding of the air underneath the ball and therefore less pressure. And by degree of physics, the ball will always move away from high pressure, and toward low pressure. Thus, a spinning ball will, during its flight, curve in the same direction as the rotation of its forward surface. For topspin, this means that the ball will inherit a downward arc in its travel.

The effect is greatly magnified by the felt cover of a tennis ball. The fuzz of the ball creates more friction with the air — better "grabbing" capability — and thus the spinning ball will pull a greater volume of boundary air around with it.

And so, since a topspinning ball will arc downward in its flight — much more so than by the effect of gravity alone — it allows a player to hit more aggressive shots and still have them find the opponent's court. Additionally, the downward bend of the ball will drive it into the court at a more vertical approach angle than a ball hit with no spin, and when the ball strikes the court, its spin and steeper entry angle will cause it to "kick" from its bounce in an apparent acceleration that results in a higher and deeper rebound. Consequently, it forces opposing players to stay further back in their own court to play the ball and to frequently receive the ball at a more uncomfortable shoulder-level height.

The effect of a backspinning ball is the opposite. In the ball's flight, the greatest friction and higher air pressure will be built up underneath the ball; therefore, the ball will want to stay airborne longer than if it had no spin. Ordinarily this would be considered a disadvantage, for a backspinning ball will "float" during its travel and have a better chance of carrying over the baseline. However, backspin can effectively be used to land a shallow shot that will "grab" the court and seemingly "back up" in its rebound, thus staying further away from an opponent who is playing deep in the backcourt. Or, if the ball is hit with good pace and low trajectory, it will tend to skid and remain low from its

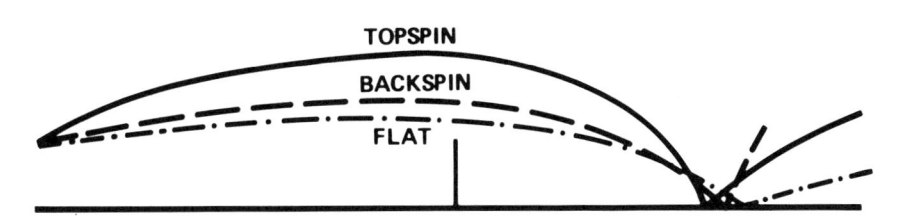

A topspinning ball can be hit to clear the net with a higher margin of safety, and its kick will compel opponents into staying deeper in their own court. A ball hit with backspin will "back up" after its bounce, making the timing for a return more unsure for opponents.

bounce, thereby coercing an opponent into hitting lunging, off-balance returns

HOW THE RACKET PRODUCES SPIN

The direction and magnitude of spin will be determined by the direction in which the racket head is traveling at the moment of impact. If the racket head is on an upward path, the ball will leave with topspin. If the racket head is moving downward at impact, the ball will be given backspin. The more emphatic the upward or downward racket path, the greater will be the spin given to the ball.

There is a widely held belief that the tilt of the racket face at impact will also have a significant effect on the spin given to the ball. In truth, the effect is minimal. High speed film analyses have shown that accomplished players strike the ball with a racket face that is essentially ninety degrees to the intended trajectory of the ball. Therefore, the angle of the racket face at impact primarily determines the loft given to the ball, while it is the upward or downward **path** of the racket at impact which provides the ball with its topspin or backspin.

HOW TO GIVE TOPSPIN TO THE BALL

Low to high. The only way a ball can be given topspin is to swing upward — low to high — so that the racket head is traveling an uphill path **before** and **during** contact with the ball. The steeper the incline of the swing, the more spin the ball will acquire. It is Newton's law of effect: the greater the impulse, the greater will be the result.

Overall, the quality of topspin produced depends on (1) the nature of the swing, (2) a controlled weight transfer, and perhaps most critically, (3) a ready state of mind to hit with the freedom which is essential for optimal results.

The Swing

To achieve the upward swing necessary for imparting affective topspin, the racket must start its foreswing from **at least a foot below the point where the ball will be contacted.** It is **not** possible to come straight into the ball and then try to lift it while it's on the strings. The racket head must be moving upward **before** it strikes the ball.

This means that the racket must be brought into the backswing lower than for a more ordinary flat groundstroke. There are two ways to do this. Either (1) take a regular unit turn and drop the racket head down during the backswing, or (2) use a loop backswing.

The more conservative preparation is to simply drop the racket head in the backswing. Let your forearm sink as you bring the racket back, even permitting some droop in the wrist. The lower you drop the racket head, the more room you'll have for generating upward momentum for the ball contact.

In the loop backswing, the intent is to whirl the racket head in a long, sweeping rainbow arc that culminates in a dramatic upward path at contact. This flamboyant

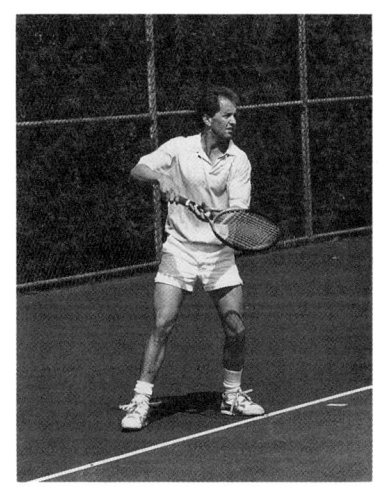

Here's the looped swing for a topspin forehand. The racket starts back . . .

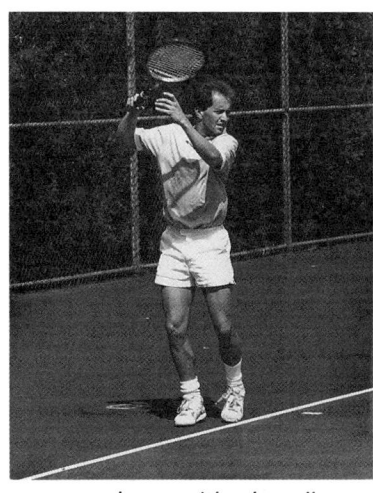

. . . and up with the elbow leading the swing . . .

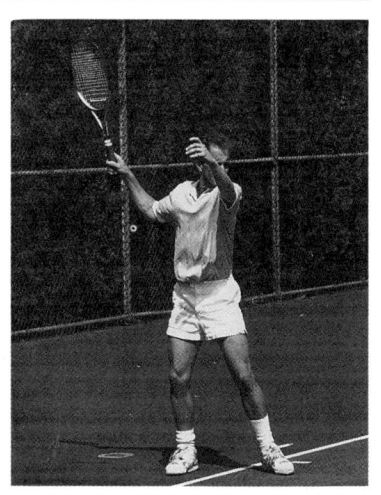

. . . to whirl the racket head around in a spherical path . . .

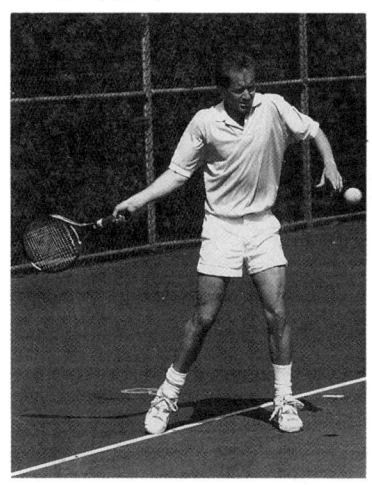

. . . . eventually bringing it below the ensuing point of contact . . .

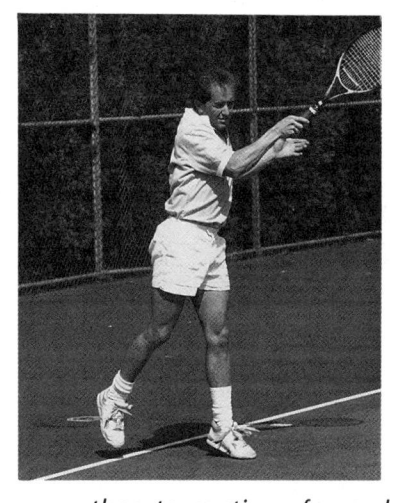

. . . then to continue forward and up into the ball . . .

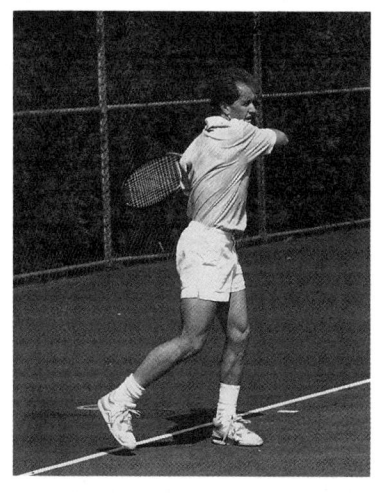

. . . finally to finish high across the opposite shoulder.

technique requires a loose forearm. Gripping the racket tightly will forbid it. Let your elbow lead the backswing, in spite of what you've always heard about not doing this. Take the racket through a long, continuous looping path, coming from behind the shoulder to swirl below waist level and then up into the ball. Keep your wrist absolutely steady as you come up and through the ball. Make it feel like the whip of the swing originates from your shoulder and forearm, not from a rolling of the wrist at impact.

Hitting topspin on the backhand side is usually more difficult. Two-handers have an advantage here, for the trailing hand can provide the useful function of propelling the racket upward into the ball with an emphatic fling that is difficult to achieve with one hand alone.

Normally, there is no loop in the backswing for a topspin backhand. Whether you have a one-handed or two-handed backhand, all that's needed is to drop the racket head down low as you prepare for the hit.

Weight Transfer

The patented suggestion of "bend your knees" has added utility for hitting topspin. By bending your knees you can more readily get your racket below the point of contact. More importantly, with bent knees you can deliver a little extra lift to the swing. Start the motion with a sensation of upward impulse that comes from your legs through your backbone, shoulder, arm, and racket.

Do not drive your weight toward the target as for a flat groundstroke. It you do, it means that your weight will be going forward while your arm is trying to go upward. Instead, make the two complimentary by giving **lift** to your whole body as you swing, generating the force from your legs upward.

The Right State of Mind

To impart topspin to a ball is not that difficult, mechanically. The biggest obstacle might be psychological. An upward swing seems impractical, and if the first few attempts send the ball into orbit, you'll be convinced of the illogic. But rip a couple of sharply descending forehands into the court and you'll be hooked.

Knowing **how** to hit topspin is the first part. The second is having a **willingness** to hit

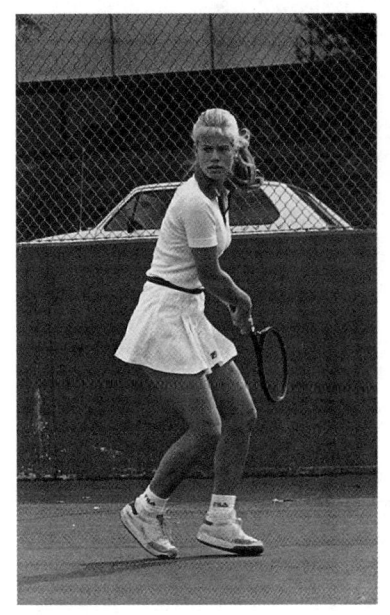

There's no loop for a topspin backhand. Just drop the racket head down . . .

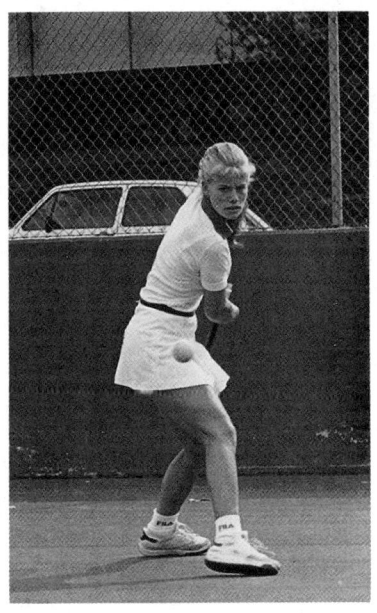

. . . and sense the buildup of energy for rotary momentum from the shoulders . . .

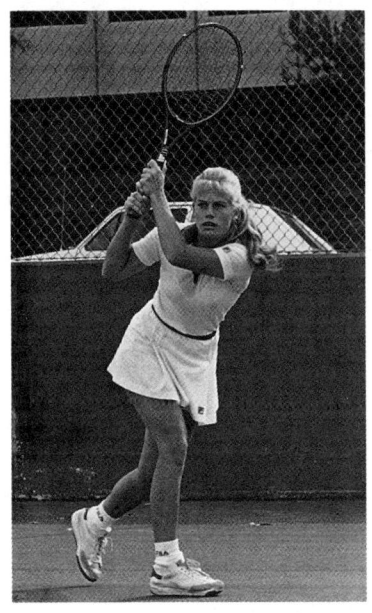

. . . the swing convincingly forward and upward without restraint, racket finishing high.

it. There can be no holding back. Your arm must be **flung** into the ball with good acceleration to produce the effect. Otherwise, the ball will simply not take the bite — it will not be compressed enough on the strings to pick up spin from the upward path of the racket. So hit topspin with a liberal mindset and a free flowing swing. Give plenty of life to the motion, and you'll become so hypnotized by its potential that you'll find ordinary flat groundstrokes mundane by comparison.

THE TECHNIQUE FOR BACKSPIN

Backspin, sometimes called underspin, is for most players easier to hit than topspin, but is not necessarily easier to control. The technique is simple: swing high to low. Bring the racket into the ball from above the point of contact. Have it moving downward at impact.

It's a mistake, however, to **chop** the racket with a dramatic downward swing. The result of such an attempt is that too much impetus is taken out of the ball and the shot will have little pace. In reality, the swing should be closer to a flat stroke to keep the racket head driving **through** the ball. It should, therefore, have both downward and forward characteristics. If there's good acceleration at impact, the ball will have a skidding, low bounce that will be tormenting for an opponent.

However, there are times when it's feasible to float a backspinning ball just over the net and have it drop shallow in the court. In such a case, the intent is to maximize the spin, so the racket should have some downward impulse with a face tilted back at contact. Not much of a swing is required for productive results, but make sure your wrist stays firm through contact.

The more you want to backspin the ball and have it drift weightlessly in flight, the more the swing must have a downward dimension with a tilt-back of the racket face. But when you want to add backspin to a normal groundstroke, the swing is only slightly downward, with little tilt of the racket face. This stroke gives the hitter a sense of **sliding through** the ball rather than one of drawing the racket down in its path.

USING SPIN IN MATCH PLAY

Because there's a net in tennis, topspin makes sense. It gives you more room on all your shots. You can lift the ball over the net with plenty of margin and have it dip into the court as if drawn by magnetic attraction. This allows you to whack your most powerful shot and watch the ball bend in-bounds instead of sailing over the baseline. Consequently, this encourages a more offensive game.

There are other merits to topspin. High-lofted topspin shots will be particularly distressing to an opponent who likes to hit aggressively, for the ball will not provide such a player with the pace that suits their game. Moreover, the rainbow arc forces opponents to stay further back to receive the ball, another frustration for a big hitter.

Tennis for Experienced Players

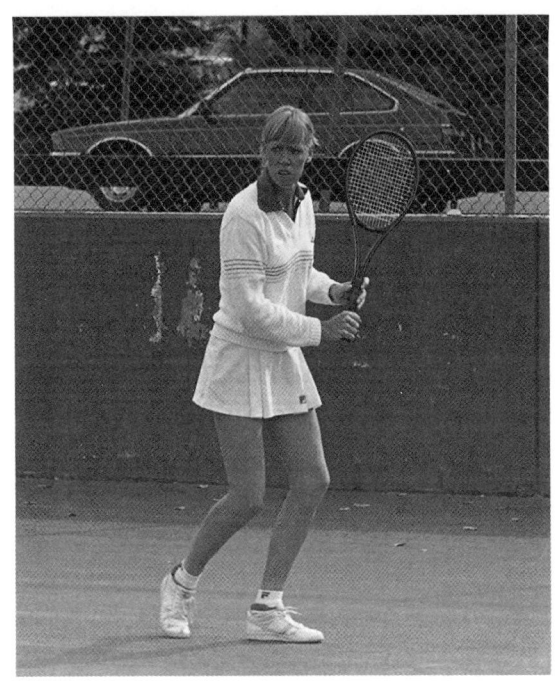

To deliver a backspinning drive to the backhand side, lift the racket head . . .

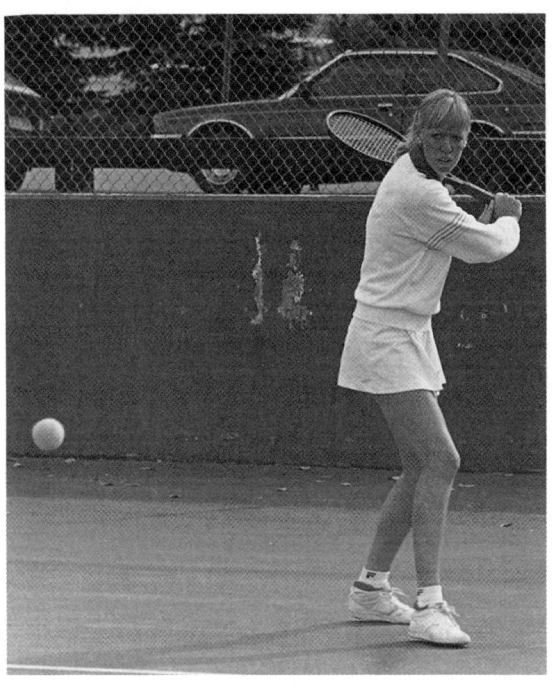

. . . into the backswing higher than the anticipated point of contact . . .

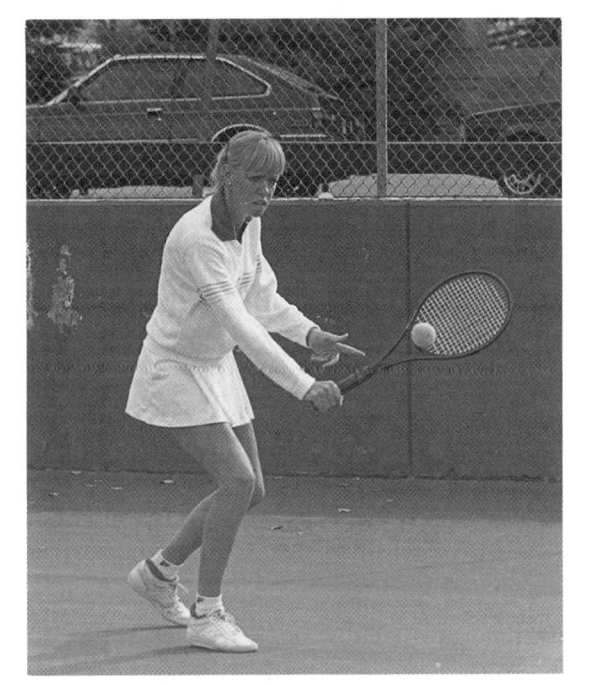

. . . then slide the strings forward and through the ball with a stroke . . .

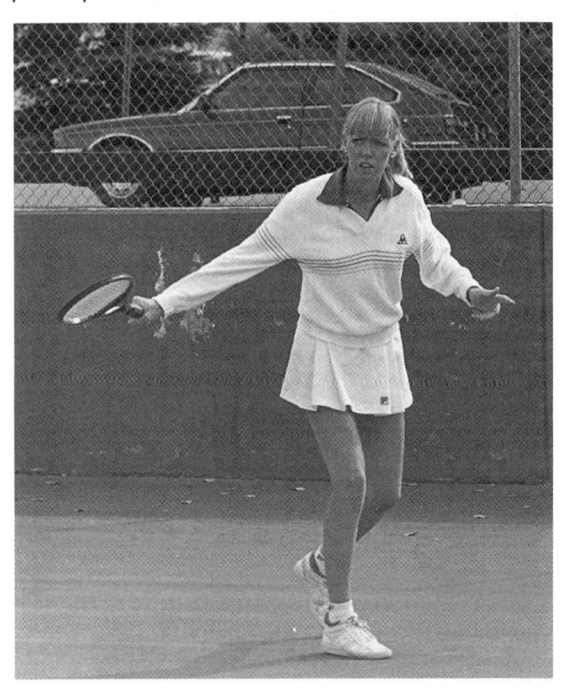

. . . that's like dragging the racket across a table top.

Hit Decisive Groundstrokes

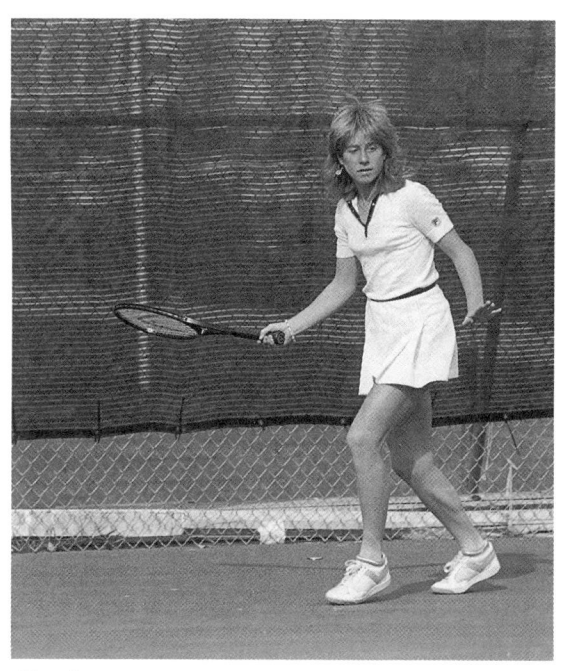

Here's a topspin forehand hit with a Western grip. Many pro players use this to facilitate racket position at contact.

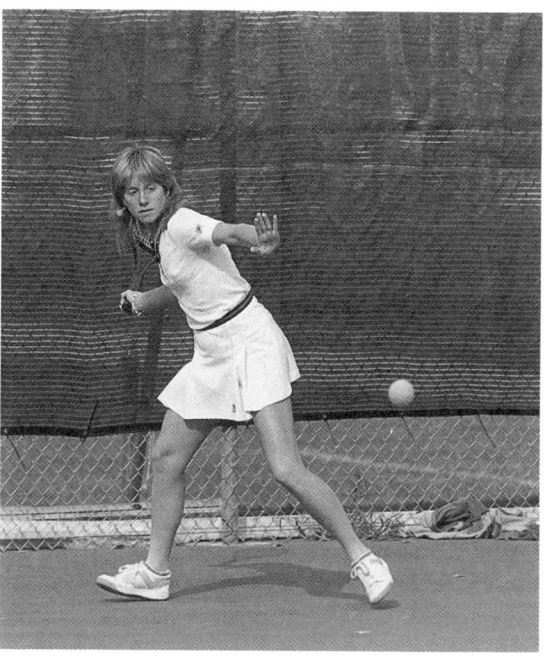

It's best used in a straight-back takeaway, as shown here, where no loop is given to the backswing.

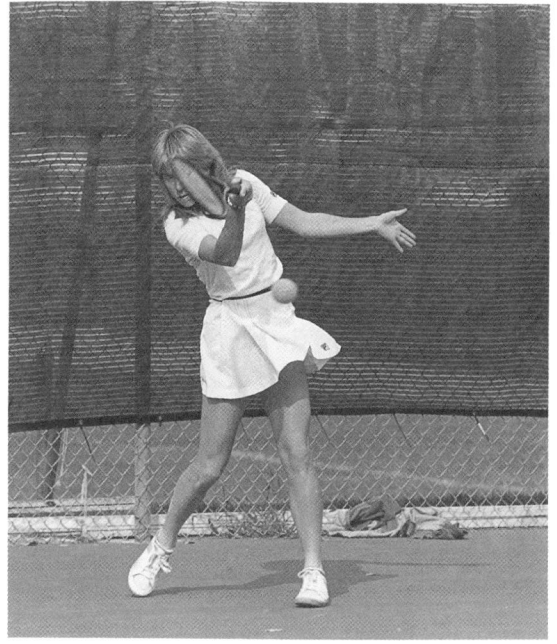

Note the open body position for contact with the ball, a factor which . . .

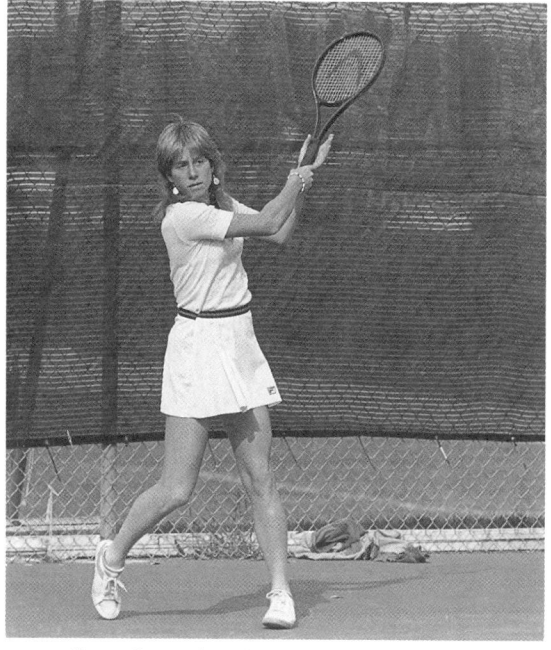

. . . allows for unhindered rotary momentum and a free, high follow-through.

Additionally, topspin is effective against an opponent who has come to the net. To attempt a flat passing shot requires needle-threading accuracy, but topspin permits you to crash into the ball and have the advantage of its dipping action. Even if you hit a strong topspin shot directly at a net player, the downward arc of the ball will make it more difficult to intercept, and the weight of the descending ball will rob the net player of their offense.

Giving backspin to a ball, though its effect is less dramatic, is a compliment to topspin. The player who can control both backspin and topspin will keep an opponent constantly off-balance. Topspin shots can force an opposing player to stay deep, and shallow backspin shots can then become surprise winners.

Backspin can also produce a deep ball without much effort, since the ball floats during its flight in apparent rebuttal to gravity. This is especially valuable when you are coerced into a defensive position, or caught on the run, or otherwise forced to hit without adequate time to prepare a normal swing.

Sliding the racket through the ball for backspin also has the effect of stabilizing the stroke, thereby producing a more solid swing that can take the sting out of a strong shot from an opponent. For this reason, forceful serves can be more effectively returned with backspin, and volleys are more durable when hit with some downward motion.

Backspin is touch. Topspin is flair. Together they make for a well-rounded player.

REMINDERS

1. For both topspin and backspin, keep the wrist firm through the hitting zone.
2. Emphatically accelerate the racket through impact for topspin shots.
3. Accelerate the racket through impact for driving backspin shots, but use touch for shallow placements of backspin.
4. For topspin, start the head of the racket at least a foot below the eventual contact point. Come up with the whole body, legs up through arm. Finish high.
5. Use an open hitting position to facilitate rotary momentum for topspin forehands.
6. Give topspin shots plenty of clearance over the net.
7. Slide the racket through the ball for backspin drives; add more downward motion for shallow placements or deep floating shots.
8. Hit topspin shots with freelanced conviction; no holding back.

PROBLEM SOLVING

Problem	Probable Cause	Solution
Not able to produce topspin	Coming straight into the ball	Drop head of racket below contact point in backswing; start low, finish high
	Wrist being used in attempt to roll racket over top of ball	Keep wrist steady throughout foreswing; no attempt to flick wrist at impact
Swing comes low to high, but still no topspin	Lifeless swing, without proper acceleration	Lengthen swing; hit with a convincing stroke; emphasize the follow-through
Ball flies too far	Racket face tilted back at contact	Keep racket face vertical for topspin; only slight tilt for backspin
	Weight stays too far back	Bring weight both forward and upward in foreswing
Ball into net	Racket face tilted over at contact	Keep racket face vertical for topspin; but tilt back slightly for backspin
	Too much chopping motion in backspin attempts	Make swing more like regular groundstroke; drive more through ball

ON THE COURT

There's a tendency to think that the wrist should "fling" the racket up and over the ball when trying to impart topspin. When watching skilled players, it appears that at the completion of their swing the wrist has "rolled over" into a palm-down finish. But that's merely a natural, anatomical response of the arm. At contact, the racket is perpendicular to the intended trajectory of the ball. Trying to give topspin to the ball by consciously rolling the wrist will dissipate some of the cumulative energy that comes through a stable wrist at impact. Besides, the ball isn't on the strings long enough to rotate the racket up and over its surface.

Check your follow-through. If you finish with the racket face down and your elbow up, you probably rolled your wrist. The ball will be listless. Take some practice balls, bounce one up into hitting height, then drive your racket, low to high, into the back of the ball with an unwavering wrist. Repeat

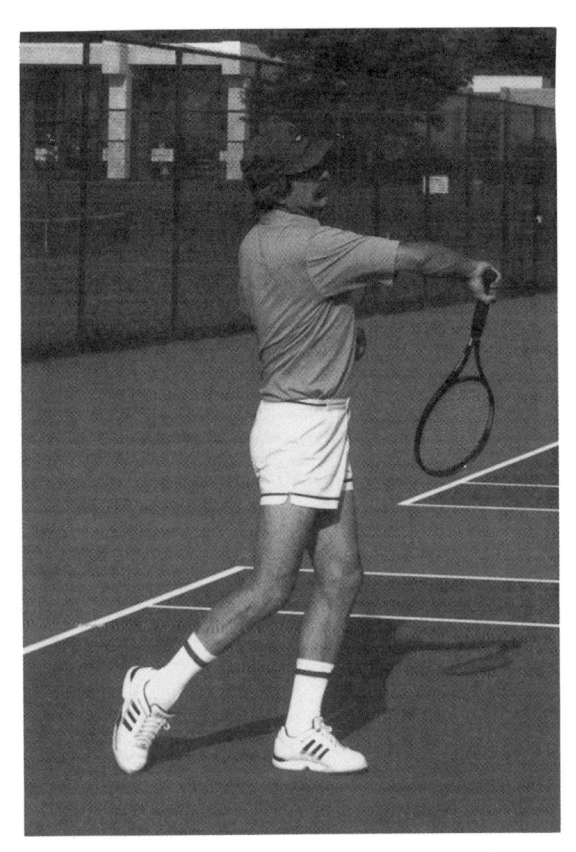

Topspin will not occur from a wrist that rolls over at contact. If your finished stroke looks like this, you lost stability in the swing.

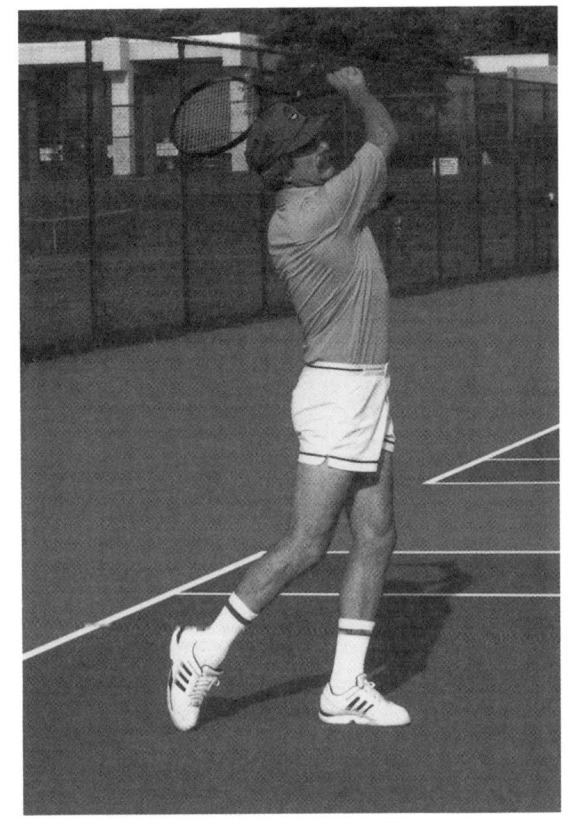

In contrast, a solid wrist at contact will transmit the cumulative impulse of the body into topspin and finish like this.

this with another ball, and another, until the resulting spin tumbles the ball end-over-end into descending flight.

Experiment with an open stance for topspin forehands. It'll give you more freedom for the rotation of your body and the upward arc of the swing. Many of the professional players hit with an exaggerated open stance to allow for upper body rotation. In so doing, they actually step away from the line of flight.

If you're not a two-hander on the backhand side, try using your spare hand to give lift to the racket as you come around, under and up through the ball for topspin. Feel uncomfortable? Releasing your spare hand before the completion of the follow-through might help, but only let go after ball contact has been made.

Extend fully through the ball on all your shots. Try to hold your racket on course. Imagine carrying the ball on the strings as long as possible. Use your racket head to say to the ball, "Go **there**!"

Give extra attention to accelerating the racket. Don't fret about hitting long. To program the feeling of acceleration, you and your practice partner could stand several yards behind the baseline, near the fence. Try to drive each ball to land on the opposing baseline.

Recognize when it's economical to give the ball spin, and when it's difficult. For example, it's troublesome to try topspin on a ball that comes to you below waist level. You simply can't get the racket down low enough. The best ones are the high "sitters" that come floating up with little pace to about chest height.

Most of all, use the practice sessions to clear your mind of any apprehension about trying to hit aggressive groundstrokes. Realize that the ball does not respond unless you let fly with a freewheeling swing. You cannot be tentative. Your arm must **fling** the racket into the ball. No holding back. Give your racket head enough speed to take it through the sound barrier. Soon you'll discover a fundamental truth about topspin: the more you accelerate the racket, the more the ball will pick up spin, and the more the ball spins the more it will arc downward in flight, and the more it arcs the better chance it has to find the opposing court. Hit ball after ball with a free-swinging stroke until you can reproduce it anytime you want without hesitation — and no fear. Then practice being humble, because the next time you play a match your opponent will keep saying to you, "Nice shot!"

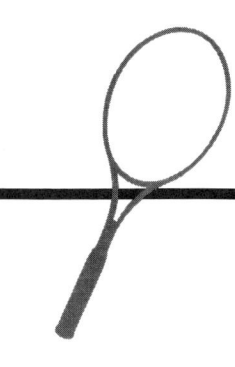

Chapter Three

Spin and Power For the Serve

Watch good servers. They **want** to serve! They **enjoy** it! They radiate confidence and hit each ball with an assured attitude that it will go in. They find serving enthralling, enlivening, arousing, and catalytic for the rest of their game.

Serving is a dynamic act. It's explosive — a free expression of power. It originates from a willing mind and a loose arm. To sense its electric pulse one must have some reckless abandon. Holding back with a conservative motion will only tighten the tendons and chords of the whole body, and the swing has a cement-arm feeling. So if you find serving troublesome, perhaps a first remedy is to clear your mind. Release your psyche. Unlock your arm. Feel unbound; untied; fluid. Fling the racket with spontaneity. Enjoy the raw pleasure of crashing into the ball with a free-spirited liveliness.

GIVE THE BALL TOPSPIN

Top level tennis requires topspin serves. The principle advantage is the same as topspin on a groundstroke: the ball will bend through a descending path in its flight to have a much better chance of finding its mark. Additionally, the definitive downward curve allows for a higher net clearance. The ball can be aggressively hit to clear the net by as much as six feet of spare room and still find its plunging way into the service court.

In contrast, with a more everyday flat serve (hit without any attempt to spin the ball), the margin for error is small indeed.

A topspin serve will also inherit some sidespin. Thus, the served ball will have not only an earthbound arc, but also some sideward slip on its journey. Then, when it lands, the topspin-produced descending arc will yield a higher rebound, and the sidespin will ricochet the ball at an angle opposite from its original flight path. Because of this exaggerated rebound action, the topspin serve is often called a "kicker," and its coercive action is quite disconcerting for a receiver.

By varying the speed and spin of the ball, topspin is suitable for both first and second serves. It can be a lethal, overpowering offensive weapon, yet at the same time an accurate staple of control.

WHAT THE RACKET MUST DO

To impart topspin to a served ball, the requirement is the same as for a topspin groundstroke: the racket must meet the ball while traveling upward — low to high. The back of the upper arm and the wrist do much of this work, flinging the racket up to clip off the backside of the ball and send it tumbling on its way with overspin.

This is a departure from the technique for a flat serve, where the racket is brought straight into the back of the ball — **flat** into the back — with the strings square to the intended line of flight and the thrust of the racket head traveling directly on that line. But for a topspin serve the swing takes the racket through a curving path to strike the ball a glancing blow. If the ball were a clock face, the impact occurs at 7 o'clock and seemingly follows through to 1 o'clock. The racket does not actually go up and over the ball, but instead kicks into the lower back of the ball while still on the upward sweep of its arched pathway. Consequently, although it may appear otherwise, the ball is actually struck before the racket has reached the extended peak of the swing.

USE A CONTINENTAL GRIP

To hit topspin serves it is imperative to employ a **Continental grip.** It is a physical law. If you use a forehand grip (common for flat serves), the upward impulse of the racket will send the ball flying off into the stratosphere. The Continental grip will compensate for the uphill nature of the topspin swing by tilting the racket face over, more square toward the target at contact, and will thankfully keep the served ball from seeding the clouds.

Check your grip often — it's easy to forget about the Continental and slip back into a seemingly more comfortable forehand grasp. Make your grip feel that you could, as you prepare to serve, more readily dribble the ball on the court with the **edge** of the racket instead of the strings.

CLOSE THE STANCE

Next, take up a serving stance that is decidedly closed. Pull your back foot around behind you, enough to make it feel you have turned too far away from the net, literally making it seem as if you must look over your forward shoulder to set your sight on the service court.

This suspiciously illogical starting position will keep the racket head **behind** the ball at contact. If you stand in a more conventional, "squared-off-to-the-net" position, it is likely that your hitting elbow would be pulled too far forward during the swing, and this, because of the Continental grip, would drag the racket around to meet the **outside** of the ball and send it off-target wide of the service court.

These two changes — the closed stance and Continental grip — will probably be disturbingly uncomfortable at first. As confirmation of their value, try a few topspin serves with a squared-off stance and forehand grip. Assuming you use the appropriate swing, the results of these trials will imprint two checkpoints in your mind before every topspin serve: closed stance, Continental grip.

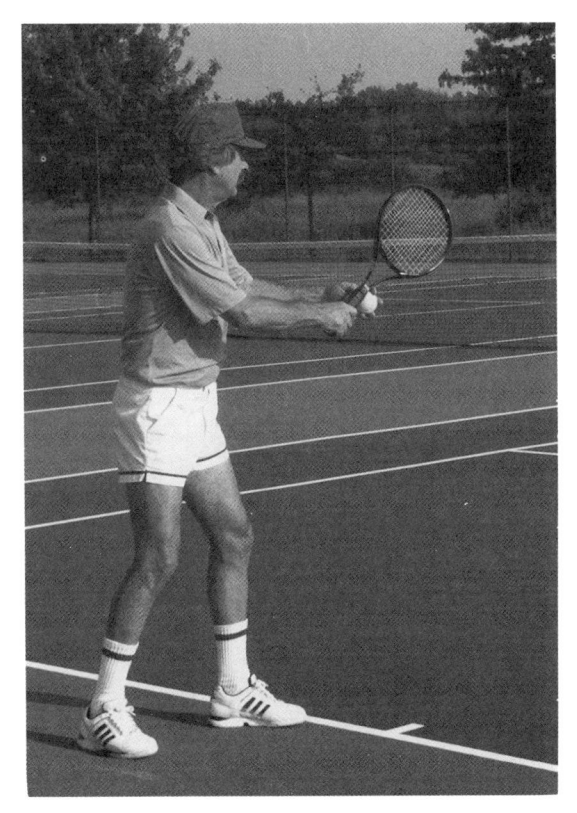

Here's the standard preparatory stance for a flat serve: body turned toward the net and the racket held with a forehand grip.

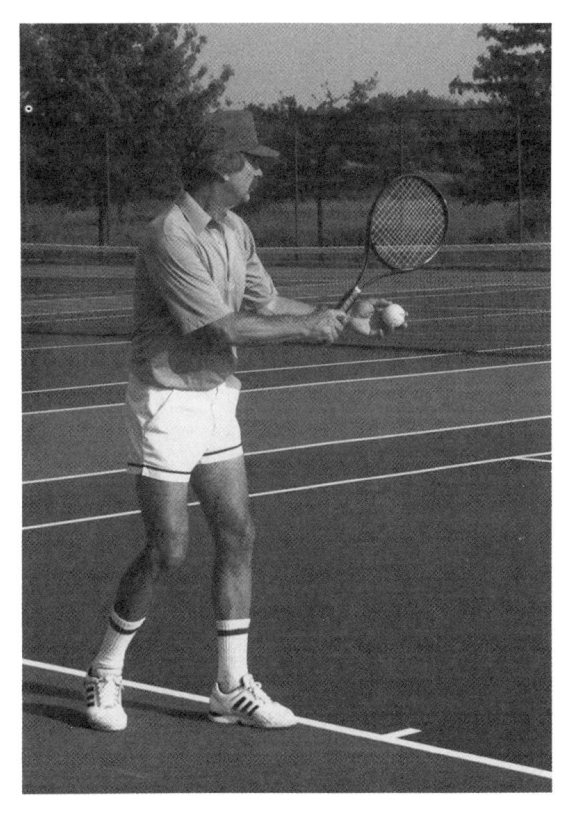

The start for a topspin serve has the body pulled around in more of a closed stance and the racket held with a Continental grip.

TOSS THE BALL FURTHER BACK

For a flat serve the ball is placed an arm's length out in front of the hitting shoulder, but for a topspin serve the ball is lifted further **back** to allow for the upward path of the racket. Make the toss so that it seems to be almost directly overhead, even though at first you'll think it's too far back.

Don't be overly concerned about grooving an exact toss. It's too easy to blame serving flaws on the toss. Just use your thumb as a guide to lift the ball to its destination. You'll find that the nature of the swing for the topspin serve has marvelous adapting properties for a fluctuating toss.

THE WINDUP

Whether you start your serve with a straight-up-and over-the-shoulder backswing

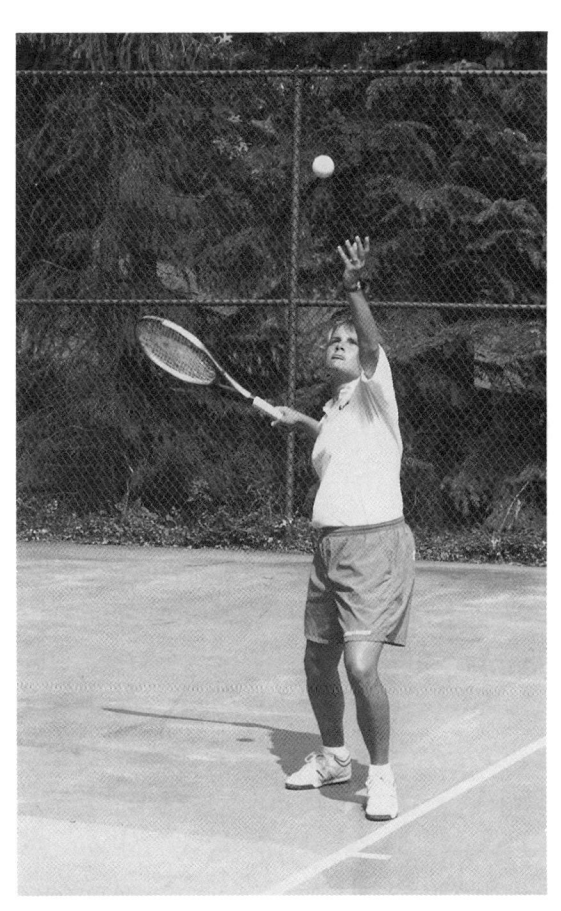

Lift the toss gently, without any flick of the wrist. Release the ball when your arm reaches unrestrained extension.

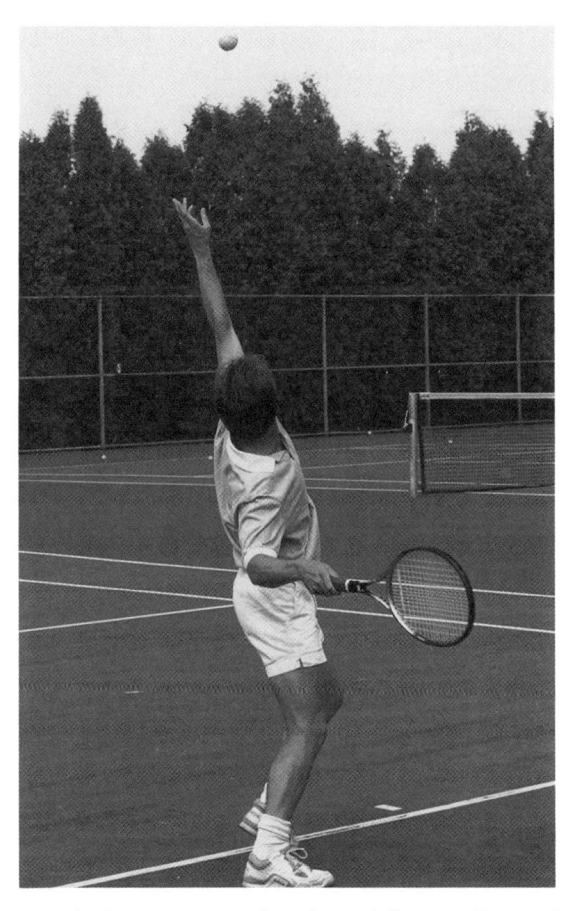

Passively open your thumb and fingers. Pretend you are trying to settle the ball onto a shelf, or releasing a bird into the air.

or an exotic double-helix pattern, the following are ingredients for successful topspins.

1. There is no hurry at the start. Until the ball is at the peak of its height, everything is slow and deliberate.
2. Throughout the serving motion, there is no stop or hesitation — only moments of gathering momentum.
3. There is an emphatic arching of the back, much more so than for a flat serve.
4. There is extra knee bend.
5. The racket drops to where its **handle end is pointing at the tossed ball**.

It's a strange contortion, to say nothing of how it feels if you have never really tried it. Properly executed, it seems that your windup has literally corkscrewed you into the ground, with your skeleton having been wrung into the configuration of a question mark. But you also feel a great sense of multiplying **power** and kinetic **energy**, for you are now a coiled up spring about to be released — a cobra ready to strike out at the helpless ball.

THE HIT

The racket inherits all your accumulated energy, and the ball becomes its victim. You've would up your physical spring and released its power into the ball.

This discharge of energy comes from the ground upward: knees rebound from their bend, the backbone uncoils, the hitting shoulder catapults upward toward the ball, and the arm thrashes up and over with the elbow unbending and the wrist adding a final vigorous snap that makes the racket feel like a whip. It's a continuous sequence of lever actions that start slowly, then finish explosively.

Remember that to get topspin (1) the racket must strike the **back** of the ball while (2) still traveling upward. Consequently, your swing must have both **upward** and **forward** impulse at contact. When accomplished, the sensation is that you've taken the racket up the back ar.d over the top of the ball to yank it down from its hanging position.

THE FINISH

A topspin serve will not drag the hitter into the court as much as a flat serve. There is more of an "up-and-over" quality to the motion, and it leaves you with an aftereffect of feeling like you've landed from a descent of a flight of stairs.

Occasionally, pause in your finished position to let this frozen follow-through give you information about what went on during the swing. If your racket has not come around to narrowly miss a whack of your knee, then you might not have accelerated it through the hitting zone, or you did not provide enough wrist snap.

ADDING POWER

At first, there may be a discouraging lack of power to your topspin serves. It can be repressing — you take a big swing, give the ball plenty of spin, and it climbs lethargically

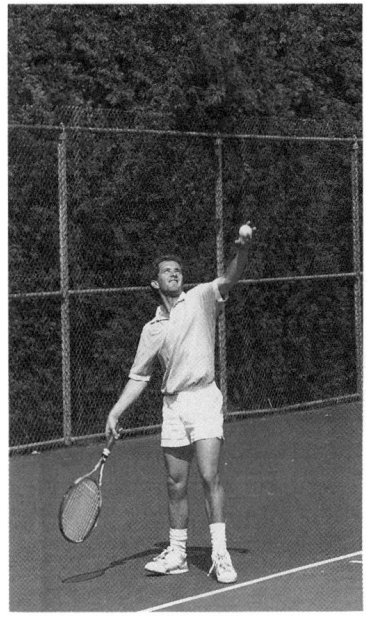

Both arms go into motion simultaneously to start the serving motion, as the toss . . .

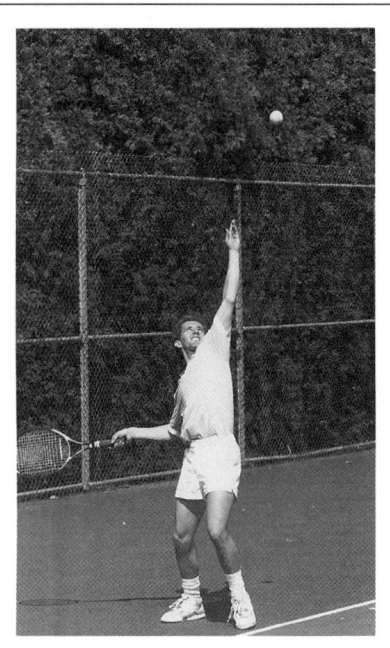

. . . for the topspin serve places the ball further back, making it seem almost overhead . . .

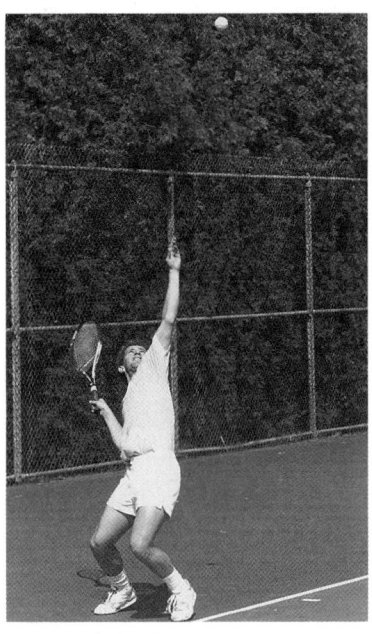

. . . while the body begins to contort into an arched, coiled-back windup and the arm takes the racket . . .

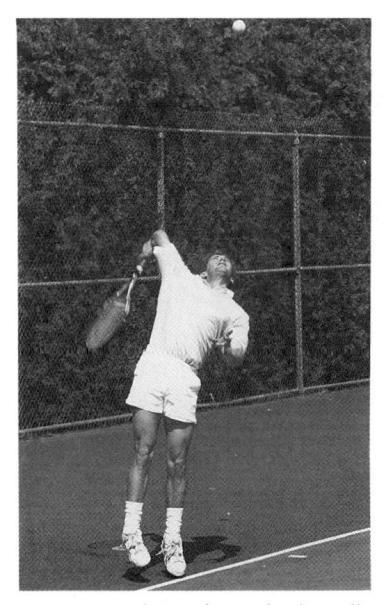

. . . around to where the handle is pointing at the ball, then uncoils spring-like for a whip . . .

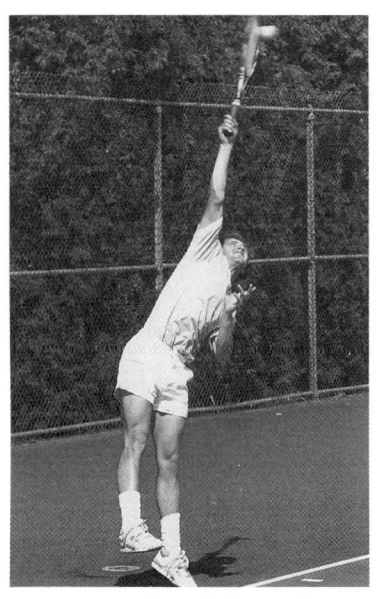

. . . upward and forward into the ball, racket snapping off the backside of the ball . . .

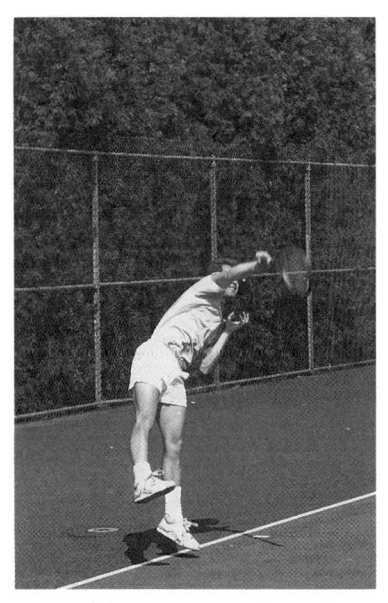

. . . with a vigorous fling of the arm and wrist that carries the racket down toward the court.

into flight. Your response might be to try serving harder by **swinging** harder. But contradictory as it might sound, the way to hit harder is to **swing easier**.

When you can't seem to hit a forcing serve, it's common to force the serve. But then the swing becomes tense; rigid in its motion. It's rather like trying to fall asleep by **forcing** yourself to fall asleep instead of relaxing and **allowing** yourself to sleep.

Watch the pros. Before serving they relax. Some shake their arm loose. Or shrug their shoulders. Maybe take a deep breath of two. They want to **calm** their body — settling it down for the rhythm of the swing. They want a loose, live arm, and they know they can't get it if their muscles are tense.

So **relax** before starting the swing. Let your body be flaccid — more so for serving than for any other part of the game. Hold the racket loosely. To help generate this feeling, hit some practice serves by holding the racket on the end of the handle with only your first two fingers and thumb.

Next, have someone watch to see if you are coordinating your weight shift properly. Your weight should be coming forward and **upward** as the ball reaches its highest point, and before the racket drops down behind you to its lowest position.

Sense a sequence to the swing. Knees-hips-back-shoulders-arm-wrist; all in that order, all uncoiling and adding their part to the whole. Use your body like a whip. Sling it into the ball.

But start slowly, deliberately. Consciously take your time at the beginning of the swing. The sequence is: slow start — fast finish.

Once underway, keep the swing going. No stops. No hesitations. The whole motion should be unbroken, without any disjointed parts. Build speed as you go. Feel like at the moment you crash into the ball your swing is still gaining momentum.

Make sure that in the swing the racket head drops down behind you — **far** down — with its handle end pointing at the ball. Have someone watch to double-check. A powerful serve comes from good racket head speed at contact. By dropping the racket low the arc of the swing is increased in length, providing more distance and time for building speed.

Make the wrist snap the final consummation of power. An otherwise well-coordinated swing will dissipate its strength if the wrist is stiff. Keep a loose wrist throughout the swing, but explode it boldly into the ball as your forearm comes up. The snap is upward, forward, and outward, bringing the racket head through a rainbow arc up over your hitting shoulder.

FIRST AND SECOND SERVES

Typical weekend players bash away at their first serve attempt and, having failed, will hit a punch-it-over-the-net-and-get-the-point-underway second serve. In truth, both serves should be hit with about the **same effort**. It's basically the **direction of the swing** which differentiates the two serves.

Speed is taken off the second ball not by slowing down the swing, but by tossing the ball further back and emphasizing the upward lift of the racket. This will magnify

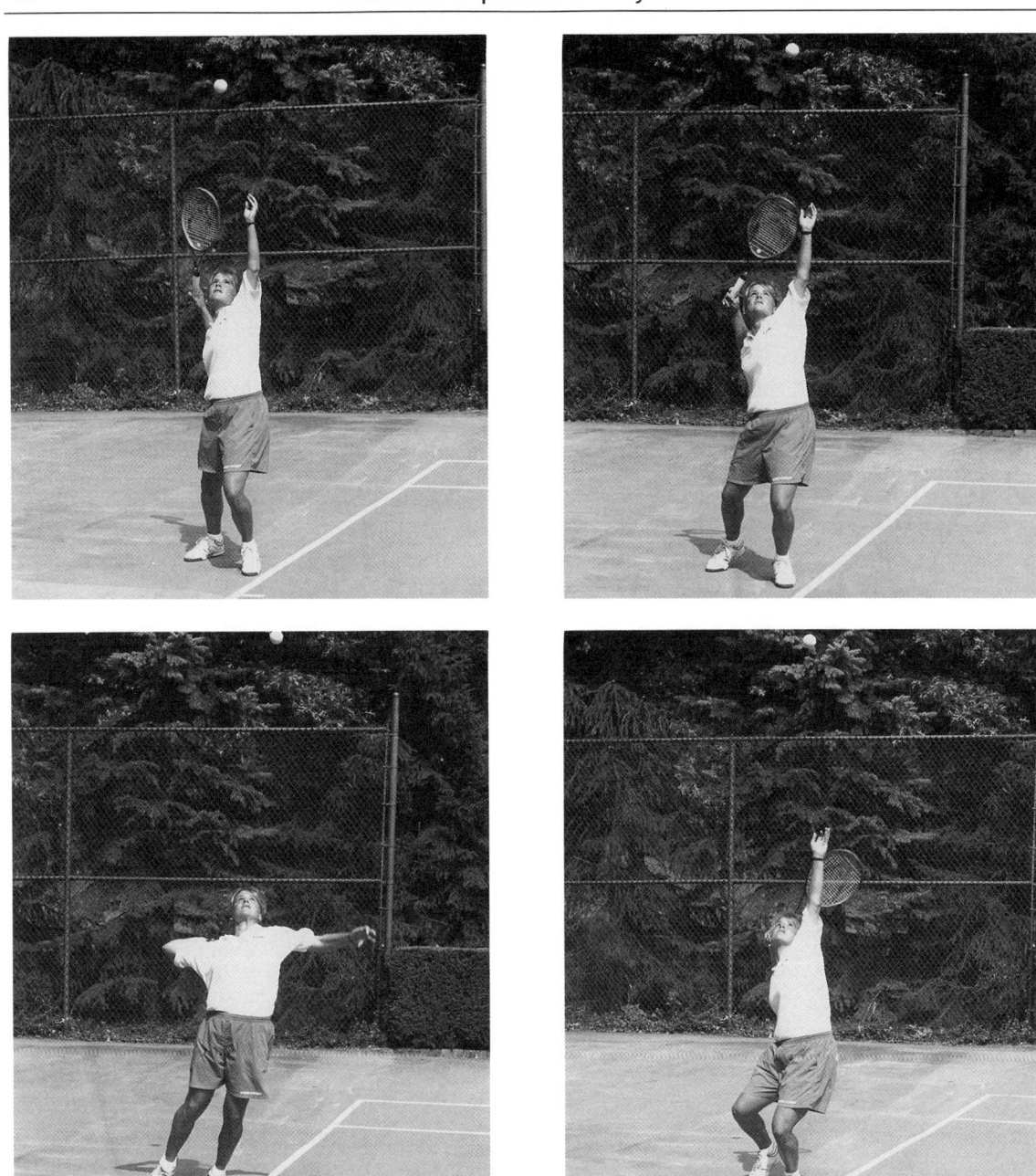

There's a subtle yet definite difference between first and second topspin serves which originates out of the toss. On the left is a first serve where the ball is tossed somewhat in front of the hitting shoulder and the body attitude is one of preparation for going up and forward. For the second serve, shown on the right, the toss is further back and there's a bit more bend to the legs to prepare for a swing which is more upward than for the first serve, but with the same explosion of energy.

the rotation of the ball and give it more bend toward the court in flight, and the slower pace will allow gravity to have more effect.

Accordingly, for the first serve the ball is tossed out in front of your hitting shoulder, and the swing motion is forward and upward. For the second serve the ball is tossed further **back**, and the motion becomes more decidedly **upward**. It's even possible to toss the ball to where it seems to be **behind** you, then swing emphatically upward and watch the ball curl into the court as if pulled by electromagnetic influence.

A key element of the second serve is conviction. It must be hit with a sense of daring, without caution in the swing. At first it will seem the ball can go only into the clouds, but soon you'll realize the same mathematical relationship as with a topspin groundstroke: more upward swing — more spin; more spin — more downward arc; more arc — more serves **in**.

ADD A SLICE FOR VERSATILITY

The slice serve is a hybrid of the topspin. It's more easily learned after having grooved the swing for the topspin.

The slice is hit with some intentional sidespin, and the airborne path of the ball is not only downward, but also sideward. The ball will swerve off to a right-handed server's left, and therefore it is more effective when hit into the far corner of the deuce court, where it will swing away from the receiver. As a result it will pull the receiver far off the court and, if not an outright winner, will open up the entire court for placement of a follow-up shot.

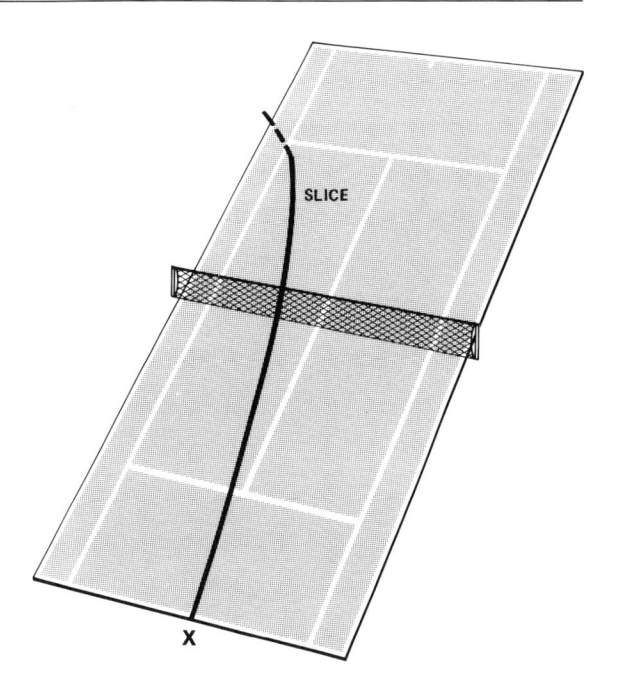

The slice serve is most effective when it's aimed at the far corner of the deuce court. Its wide rebound will send the receiver racing off the court; therefore it presents an opportune time for following up to the net to quickly volley any return into the empty court.

Left-handers have a bonus. A left-handed server can swing the ball wide in the advantage court, not only pulling the receiver off the court but also attacking the presumably weaker side. It's the best time to follow the serve up to the net.

To hit a slice, toss the ball more out to the side. Swing the racket somewhat "out and around" the ball, but still with good upward impulse. Imagine hitting the lower outside corner of the ball. Let you elbow be more of a lead in the swing, racket trailing behind, and this will emphasize the outward circular path of the racket head.

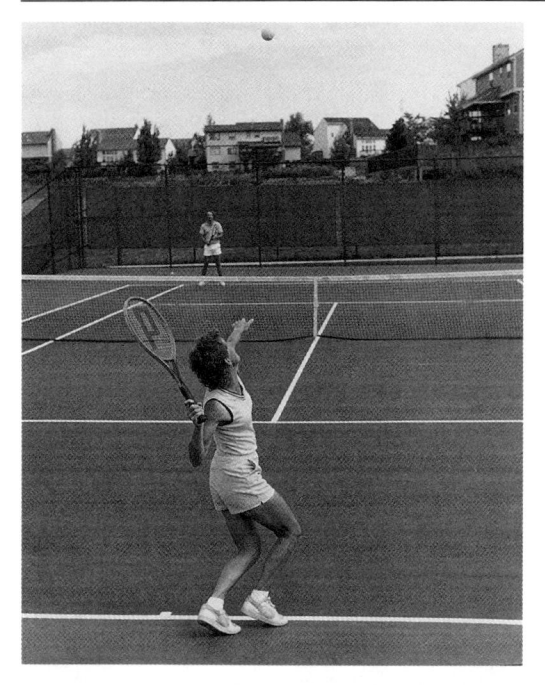

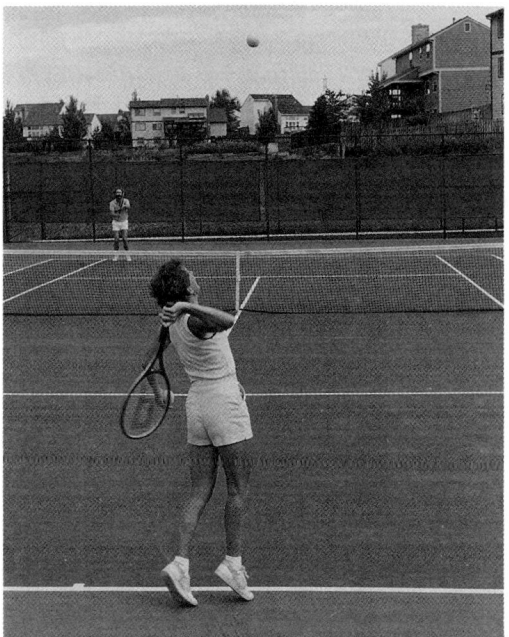

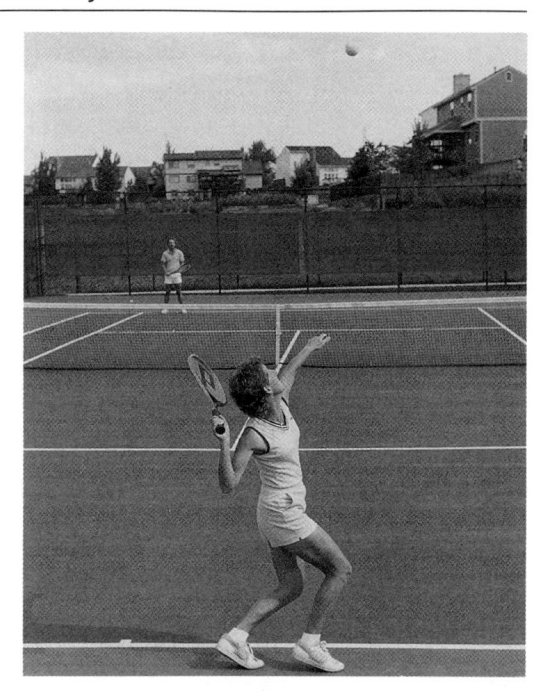

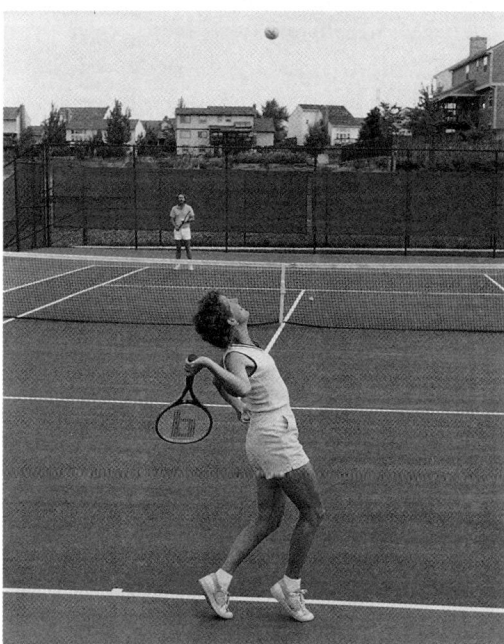

The nature of the slice serve is more clearly seen when compared to a flat serve. Here (and on the following page), in the photos on the left, the server delivers a flat serve. Note that the momentum of the swing is forward, with the racket head flat behind the ball at the moment of contact.

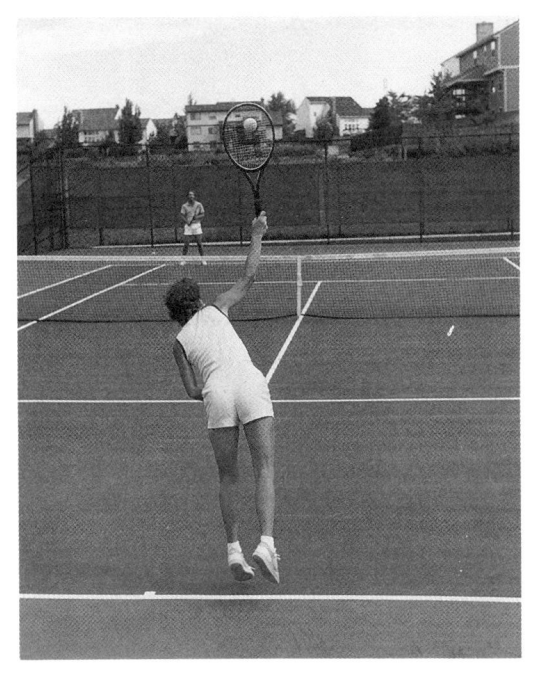

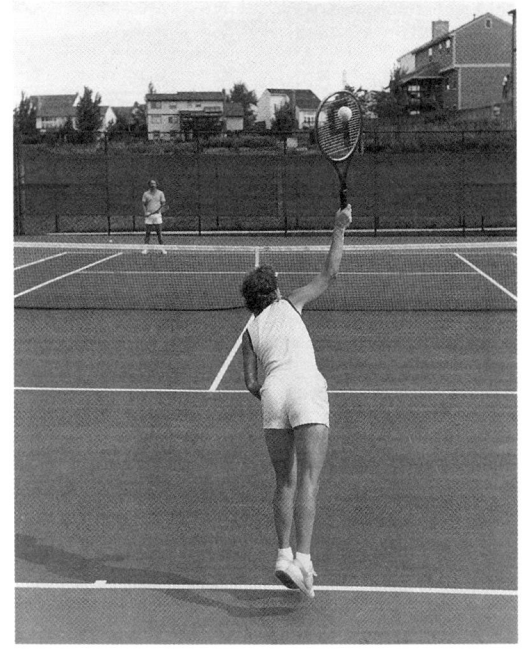

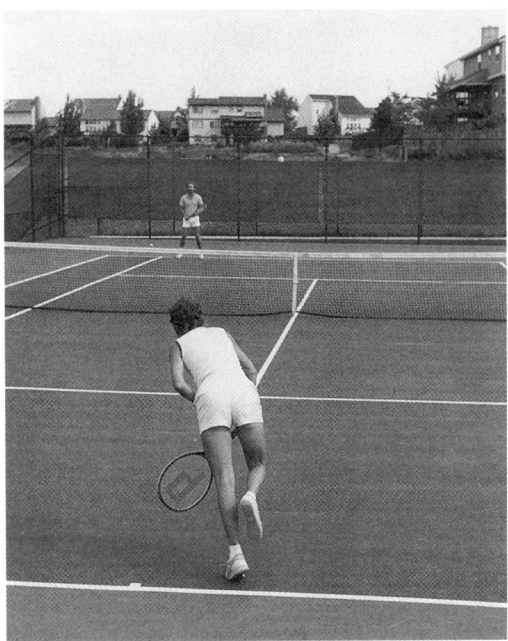

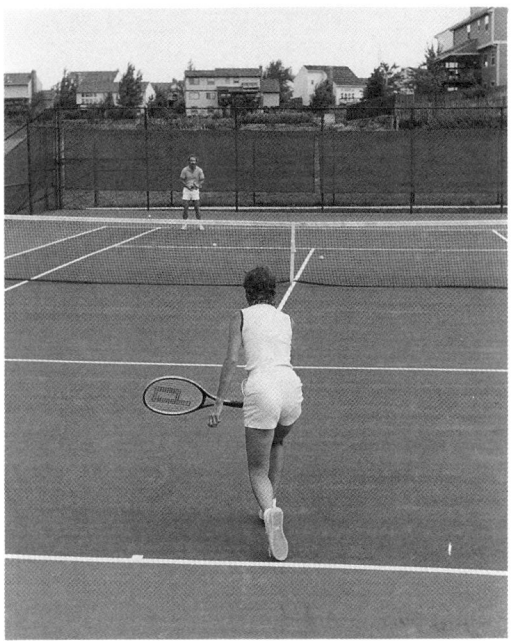

A slice serve is demonstrated here (and the previous page) in the photos on the right, starting with a more pronounced coiling and arching of the back for the swing. At contact the racket head is on its way around the lower outside corner of the ball, and this whip of the swing brings the racket into a follow-through which is more to the left of the server than for a flat serve.

REMINDERS

1. Serving is a dynamic, explosive, whole-body act. Create a picture of it in your mind before starting.
2. Relax your whole self. Let your arm go limber. Make it feel like spaghetti.
3. Close the stance. Take a Continental grip.
4. Spiral yourself into a coiled windup, racket head dropping behind your back, handle pointing skyward.
5. Unwind sequentially toward the ball, legs up through the arm, finally a vigorous wrist snap.
6. Make the whole motion continuous, rhythmical.
7. Fling the racket into the ball, whip-like.
8. Start slow — finish fast. Build speed throughout the swing.
9. For topspin hit the **back** of the ball, racket still moving upward.
10. For slice serves hit the lower outside corner, racket moving up and out.

PROBLEM SOLVING

Problem	Probable Cause	Solution
Serve too long	Ball tossed too far back	Lift heel of tossing hand, toss further out
	Pushing at ball	Emphasize whip of arm and snap of wrist
Serve into net	Ball tossed too far out in front	Toss further back; swing more up
	Failure to transfer weight	Emphasize push off back foot
No power	Failure to coil shoulders in backswing	Take racket back with a unit turn, much as in preparation for a forehand
	Failure to arch back in windup	Crank body into a coiled, spring-like windup
Still no power	One-piece swing	Uncoil sequentially upward and forward into ball; legs first, arm and wrist last
	Insufficient whip in swing	Loosen forearm before windup; keep a whiplike feeling throughout swing
Only minimal ball rotation	Not dropping racket down far enough in backswing	Drop racket to where the handle is pointing to tossed ball
	Not snapping wrist	Hold wrist back, release at last second
Still not enough topspin	Swing momentum going too forward	Emphasize the upward character of swing, especially lifting elbow up
	No spring to body	Bend knees more in windup
Too much sidespin on ball	Racket coming too far around outside of ball	Stay sideways to net as long as possible in serving motion
	Elbow too much of lead in swing	Hold elbow back as foreswing starts, then lift elbow emphatically upward

ON THE COURT

Think of a javelin thrower. The body uncoils dramatically, the arm extends fully up and forward at the moment of release. You can almost **feel** the power.

Strong serves need that same explosive release of energy. During practice, let fly with your most exertive efforts. Turn the throttle to full speed.

Spend alot of practice time hitting second serves. It'll be of direct benefit for honing these follow-up serves and will indirectly help the first serve by promoting a free-swinging motion. Develop a second serve that will rarely fail under pressure. This will be a great

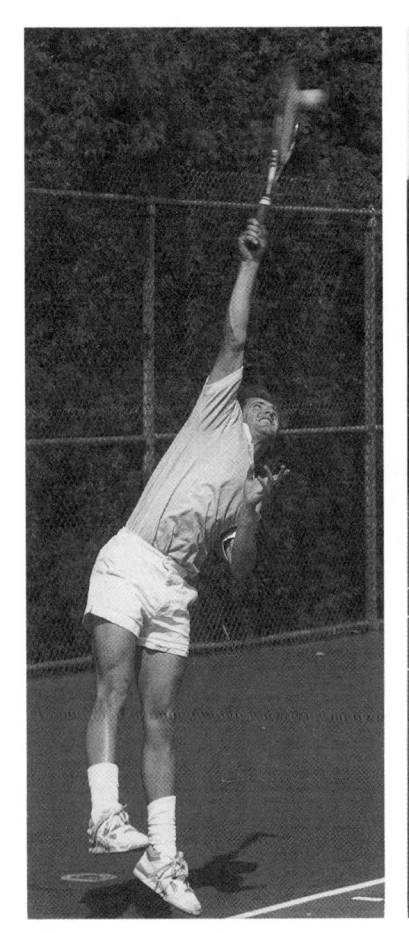

Give your practice serves lots of explosion. No holding back. CRUSH the ball on your strings.

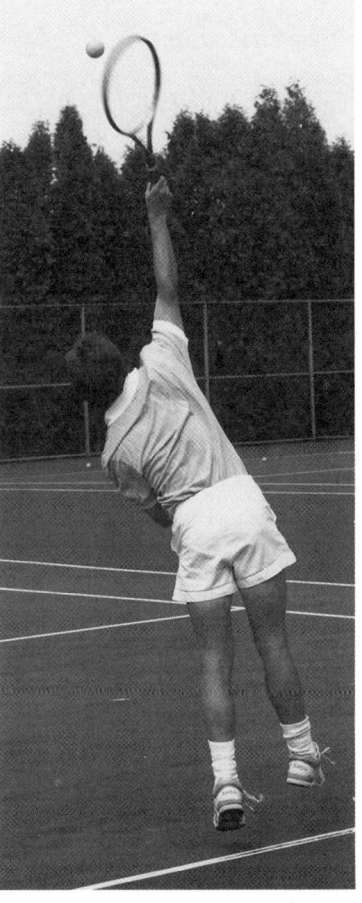

Fling the racket, whiplike, into the ball with free-wheeling abandon. Feel explosive energy going into the ball.

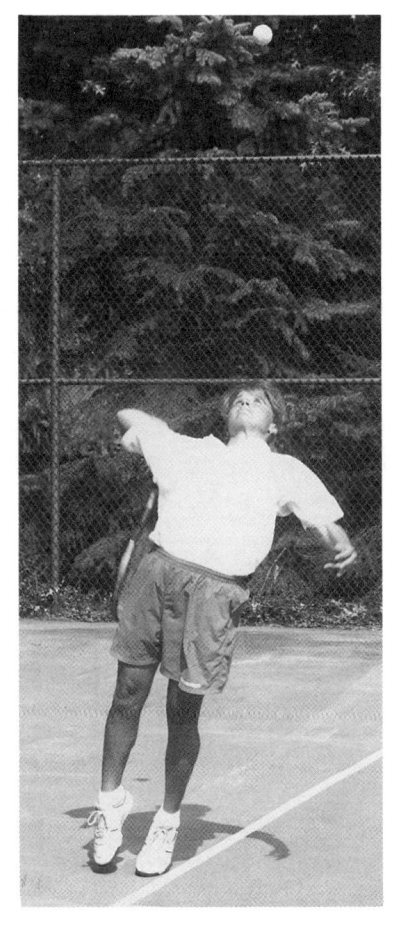

When practicing second serves, emphasize the drop of the racket to point the handle skyward at the ball.

psychological edge in match play where you could otherwise become nervous and frustrated with the progress of the contest.

Now is the time to experiment. Pull your grip around toward a backhand. Hit some topspin serves. Pull it around even more. Keep turning it toward the backhand until you start hitting off the edge of the racket. The closer you can get to a backhand grip, while still hitting the ball solidly, the more spin the ball will acquire.

You must compliment this, however, by emphasizing the upward thrust of the racket. Try to drop the racket head as low as you can in the windup, arriving eventually with both the handle of the racket and your **elbow** pointing upward toward the sky. Then feel like you're swinging up and into the ball by lifting your elbow, arm coming up and over. Focus especially on the upward thrust of your elbow. Think **up** before you swing. Try extra knee bend to help prime the upward thrust of your swing, particularly for second serves. Imagine sitting down in a chair as you take the racket into the backswing

Don't worry about too much bend, there isn't enough time to get too low.

Eventually you'll realize the second serve is much like the first. You can hit all-out on both attempts. It's the direction of the swing, not the effort, that is different.

Experiment also with your stance. Second serves are often facilitated by a very closed stance, whereas slice serves need more of a square stance.

Keep exploring new ways to hit the ball. The serve is probably the most individualized part of tennis. Everybody must find their own best style — within reason of physics.

The serve should actually be the easiest stroke of all. It's the one stroke you fashion for yourself, as an action rather than a reaction. Everyone can develop their own natural rhythm, and their own pacing to become a smoothly functioning tennis machine. Then, when everything has fit together into a self-lubricating motion, you'll believe you are responsible for those statements about the serve being too much of a dominating factor in tennis.

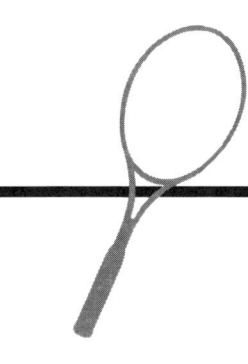

Chapter Four

Designed Service Returns

The return of serve is the most neglected phase of tennis. Rarely is it ever practiced, or ever even **thought** about. But statistics compiled in professional matches show that the service return actually influences the outcome of more points than any other single stroke, including the serve itself. At all levels of play, it can neutralize a big serve and provide the receiver with a great psychological advantage.

Much of the success in returning serve is dependent on reflexes. There's little time when the ball is approaching at tyrannical speed. So the receiver must sometimes block, chop, chip, slap, or punch the ball back. Anything to make the server play another ball. It is the first objective of receiving serve, and sometimes the only one needed. But from a tactical viewpoint, there are other things a receiver can do to take the offensive.

WHERE TO STAND

When receiving serve, take up a position in the middle of the widest possible area into which the server can hit. But consider that most players will have more difficulty swinging the ball wide into the far corners than hitting up the middle. Also, if you have a stronger side, you may want to give more room to that side.

How far in you stand depends on the talents of both you and the server. Staying

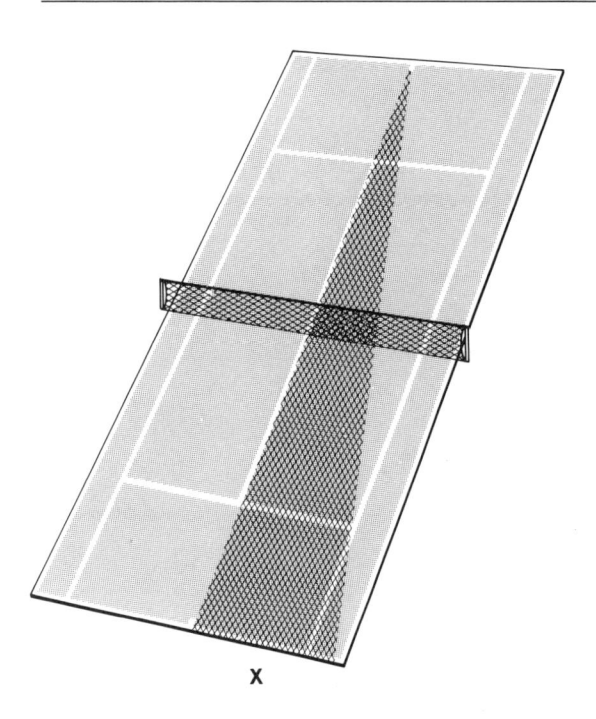

Generally, it's most economical to stand in the middle of the widest angles the server has for placement, and as far in as you can while still being confident that you can handle the best the server has to offer.

back gives you more time to set your sights on the ball, but this also provides the server with more opportunity for hitting out of your reach to either side. It also gives the server more time to charge the net and get into effective volleying position.

Consequently, it's best to be in as far as you can and still feel confident in being able to hit under control, for three reasons: (1) any spin the server gives to the ball will have less time to work it's effect, (2) you'll not be drawn as far off the court by wide serves, and (3) there will be less time for the server to approach the net.

GETTING READY

As the server prepares to hit, remind yourself to:

1. Hold the racket loosely. If you're really tense, spin the racket a few times or open your hitting hand completely while you take the weight of the racket in your other hand.
2. Hold the racket in front, pointed at the server so that it can be quickly drawn to either side. Rest your elbows comfortably in front of your hips.

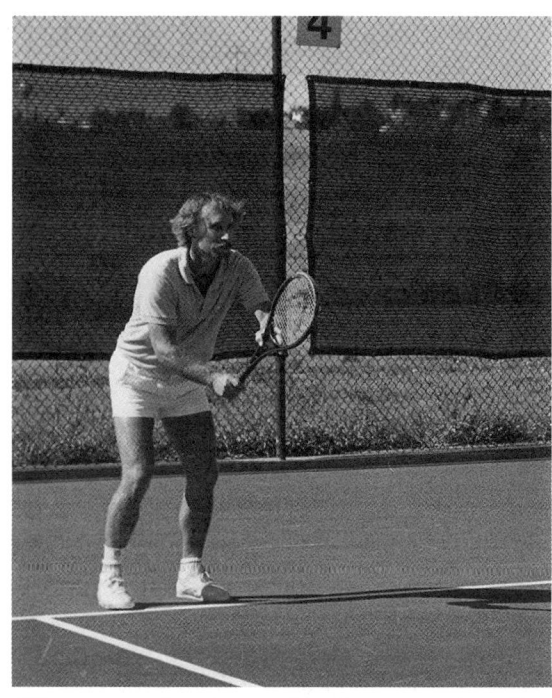

*When preparing to receive the serve, be alive, alert, responsive. Keep the racket forward, held loosely, elbows in front of hips, with weight ready to move **forward**. Be primed to pounce on the ball, cat-like. Have all your senses wide-awake, building them to peak alertness just as the ball is served.*

3. Have your weight **forward**, on the front of your feet. Pretend that a wedge has been pushed under your heels. Keep a flexed body and a low center of gravity.
4. Look at the server's feet. A closed stance indicates a topspin serve is likely. A more open stance means a slice.
5. Zero in on the ball like adjusting a pair of binoculars. First see the whole scene — server, racket, ball — then narrow in on the ball as it reaches the peak of the toss. Rivet your focus on the ball to get you into a momentum of readiness.

WHEN THE BALL IS ON THE WAY

Abandon any natural tendency to backpedal in anticipation of a hard serve. Instead, you should be primed to move **forward**. Be ready to go **at** the ball! **Pounce** on it! Meet it **early**!

Taking the ball as early as you can will keep you from being pulled off the court by a wide serve. You have less court to cover — less distance to go to intercept the ball. And by moving **at** the ball, you'll be able to put more weight into the return.

So don't step sideways. Turn your shoulders quickly, get the racket back, and make your first step **diagonally forward, toward the ball**. Keep thinking **early** as the ball is about to be served.

See the ball twice: once as it comes off the server's racket, and again as it comes off the bounce. Refocus as the ball bounces. Notice how much bigger the ball gets after the bounce.

WHEN THE BALL ARRIVES

There's little time. Take an **abbreviated** backswing, **tighten** the grip, and **thrust** the racket into the ball like hitting a strong volley stroke. Don't take the racket behind you but keep it, relatively speaking, behind the ball.

There is nothing tricky or fancy about returning a big serve. Borrow the power that is already on the ball. Keep a firm wrist, and shorten everything about your swing. Make it compact, but solid.

On really hard serves you can use your non-hitting hand to help push the racket back for a forehand or pull it back for a backhand. If the ball is hit directly at you let self preservation take over. Push off one foot, quickly turn your upper body to open your shoulders and pull them **away** from the ball. Brace your grip extra firm for the impact.

Especially on the backhand side, try beveling the racket back a bit and bringing it into the ball slightly downward. In this motion you will use the stronger muscles on the back of your arm, and this, coupled with a hammerlock grip, will steady the racket head. Additionally, the downward motion of the racket will give a little extra thrust to take the pace off the ball and turn it around. Be careful not to make this a "chopping" motion. Rather, **slide** the racket through the ball.

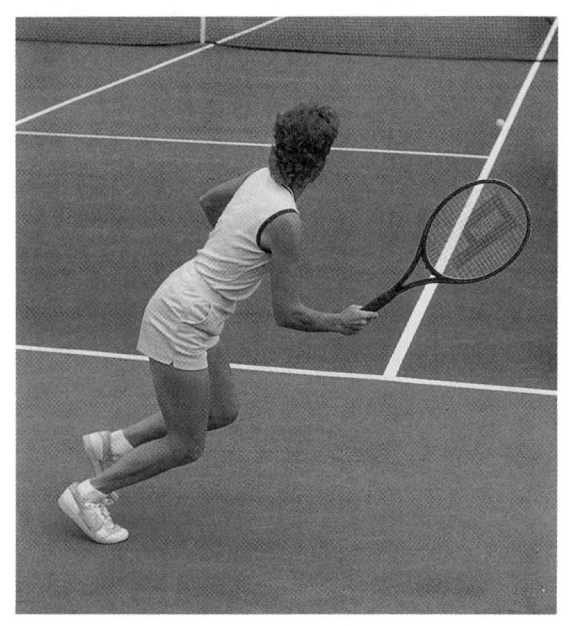

Here comes a wide serve, and the receiver has turned to chase the ball . . .

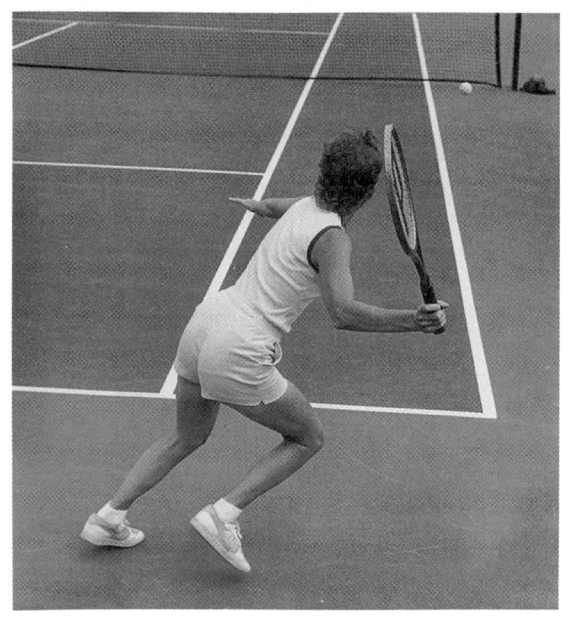

. . . by incorrectly running parallel with the baseline . . .

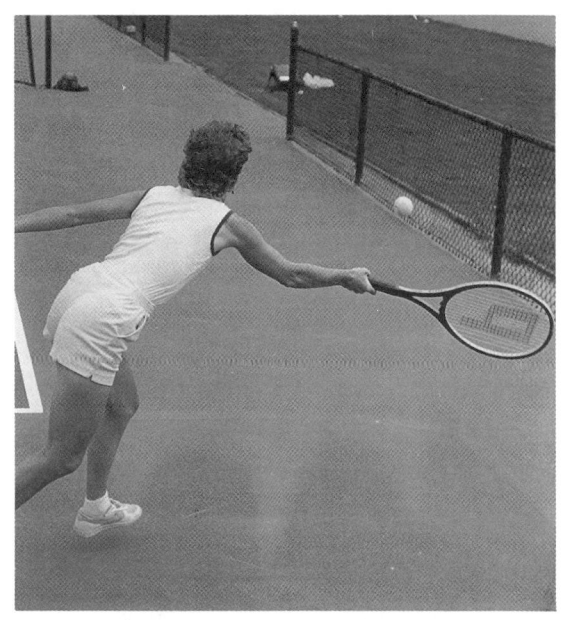

. . . and thus being compelled into a strictly defensive return . . .

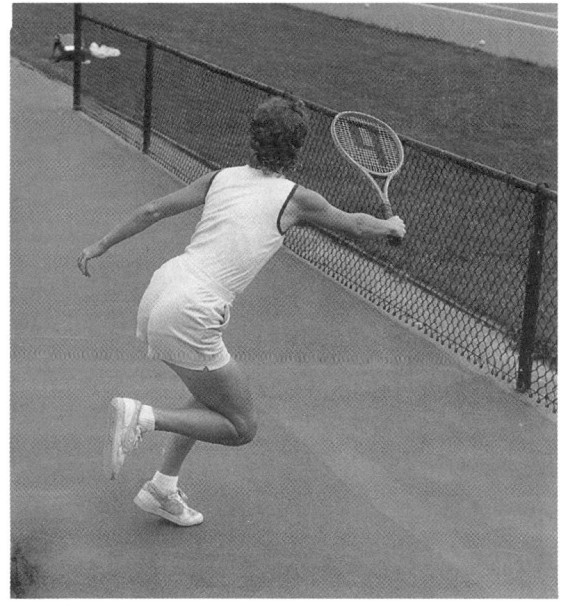

. . . and being pulled too far off the side of the court.

Designed Service Returns

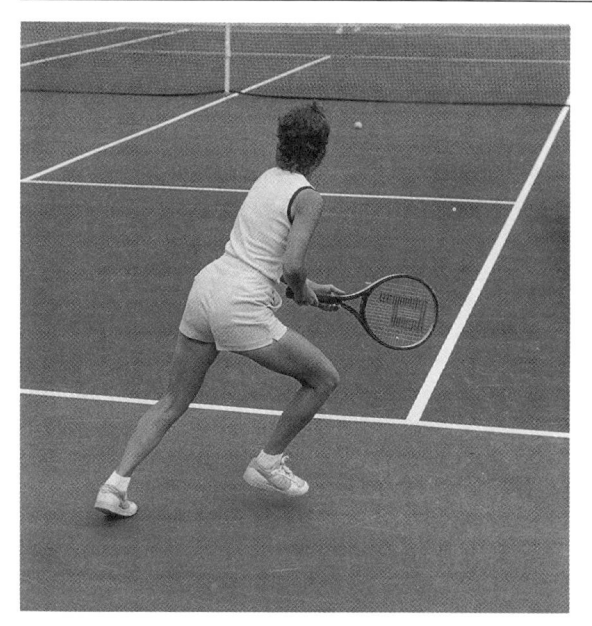

Here's another wide serve, but this time the receiver goes 90 degrees to the flight of the ball . . .

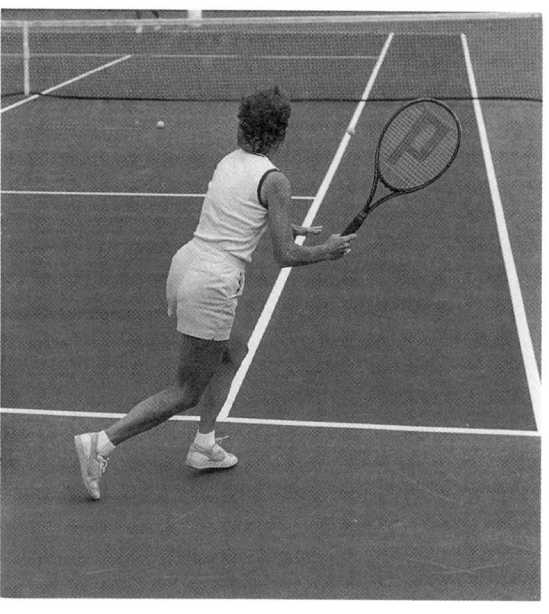

*. . . thus moving **diagonally forward** . . .*

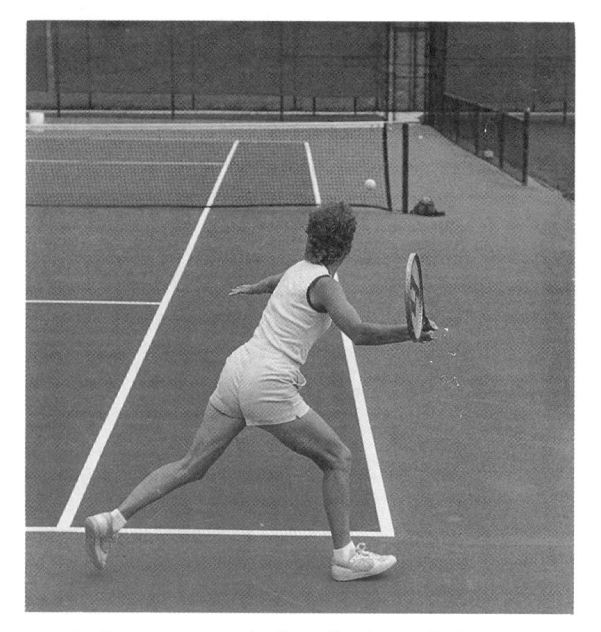

. . . to intercept the ball earlier in its flight . . .

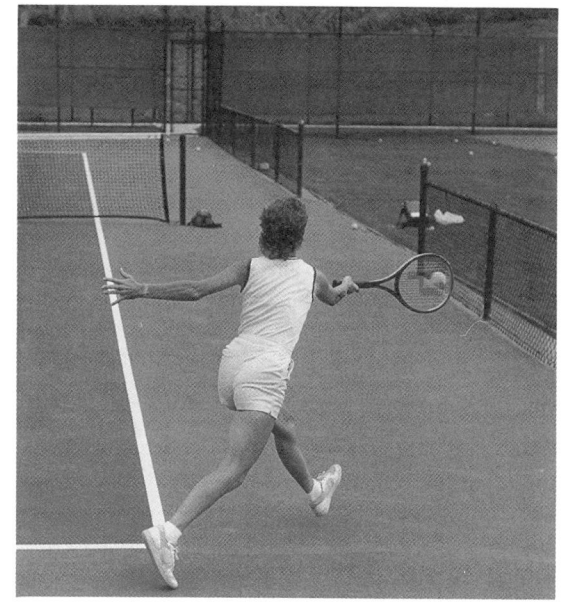

. . . and avoid being pulled as far off the side of the court.

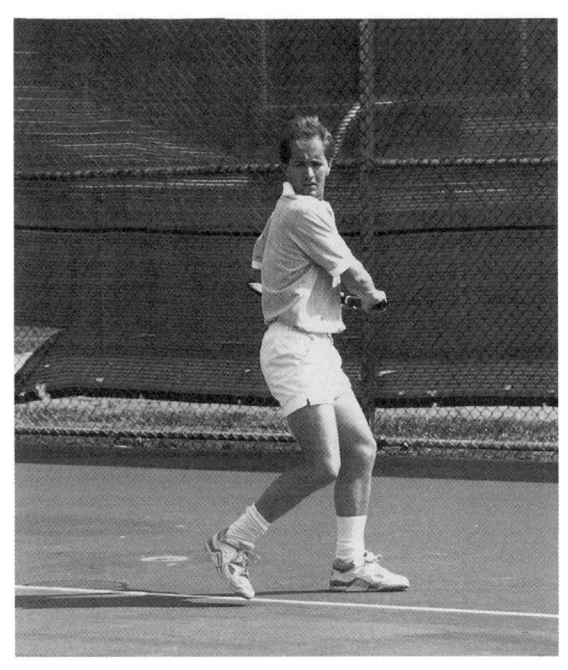

When receiving a forceful serve, get your shoulders turned as quickly as possible . . .

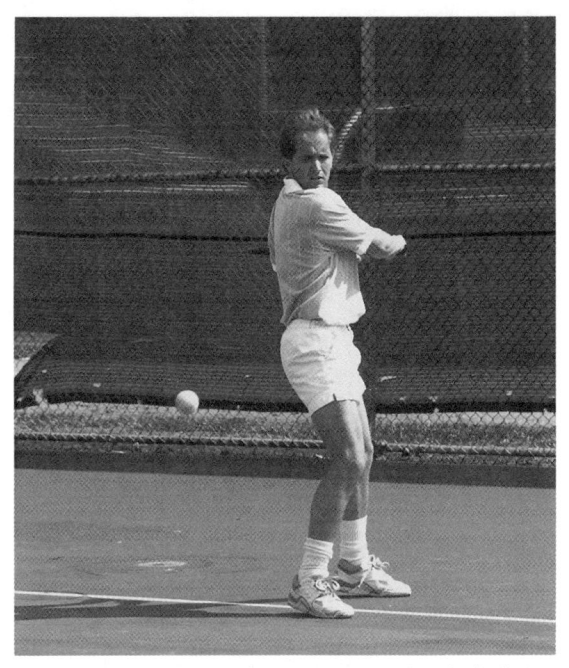

. . . using your non-dominant hand to help bring the racket into a shortened backswing . . .

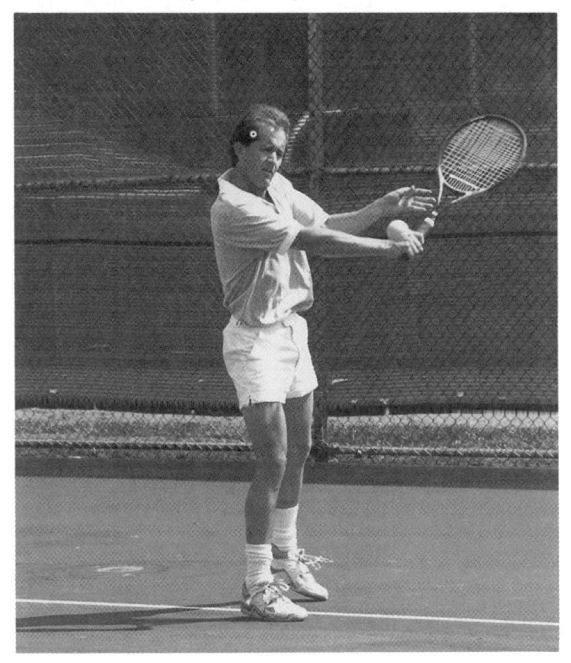

. . . then return the ball with a firm downward and forward sweep of the racket head . . .

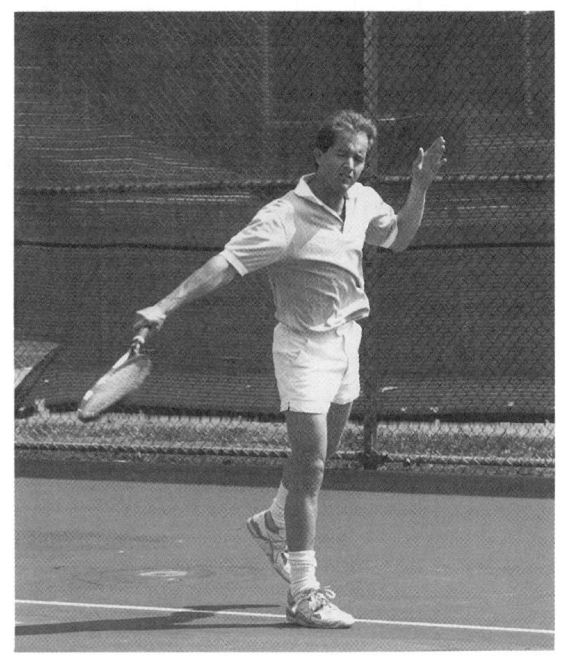

. . . keeping the wrist and forearm solid throughout the stroke.

WHERE TO SEND THE BALL

The server's advantage disappears quickly if you can return the ball with purpose. Don't think of trying to launch a missile, but have some placement objectives in mind.

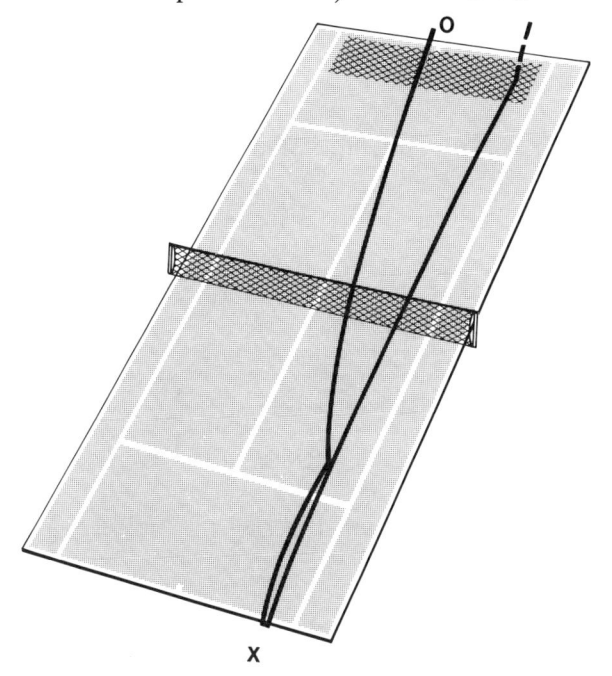

When the server does not approach the net following the serve, the best place to send the return is deep, preferably to the server's weaker side.

If the server does not rush the net, the return should be hit deep, preferably to the weaker side so there's less chance of being hurt by a strong follow-up shot. Be cautious about trying to chip a short return just over the net, because (1) it's a difficult shot to transact if the serve has plenty of pace, and (2) most players finish off their serve having been pulled in front of the baseline where they are already in a better position to retrieve a shallow placement of the return. Consequently, a deep return will coerce the server into backing up to take the ball after the bounce (very few players will attempt to hit the ball on the fly from near their own baseline). Thus, you take away the momentum the server would otherwise maintain as an aftereffect of the serve.

If the server comes up to the net, the placement must be kept low, landing the ball somewhere near the intersection of the sideline and the service line. That way the server will need to bend low and lift the ball up to clear the net, and therefore the ball will need to be hit more defensively.

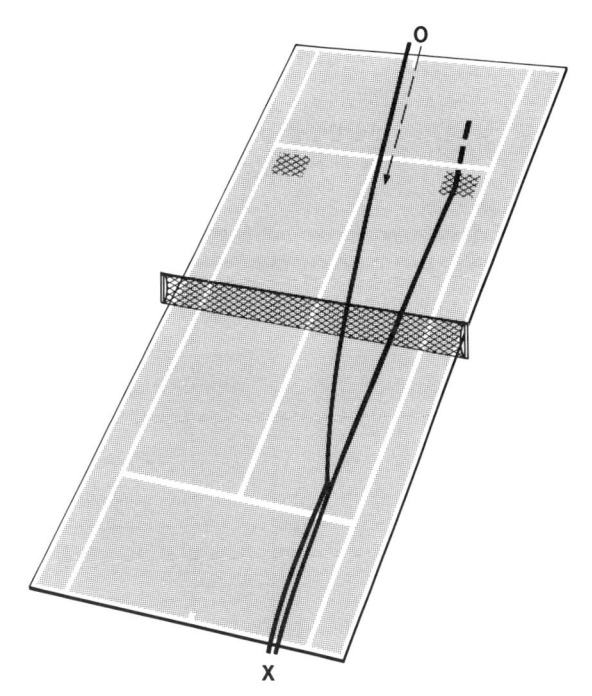

When the server charges the net following the serve, the return should be hit to land on either side of the server near the intersection of the service line and the sideline.

It is commonly stated that the best place to return the ball against a net rusher is at their feet. But such placement keeps the ball in front of the server, within easy reach. Instead, it's infinitely more effective to make the server lunge for the ball by laying it off to the side. Often, this will win the point outright.

REMINDERS

1. Think positive things as you await the serve. Keep your mind actively engaged on what you will do.
2. Keep everything simple.
3. Be ready to move **forward**.
4. Be ready to move **early**.
5. The harder the serve, the more compact the swing must be.
6. Move **at** the ball. Put life into your legs.
7. Hit the return aggressively, but not recklessly.
8. Keep a solid, firm wrist.
9. Focus intently on the ball as it comes off the server's racket, and have a "scrambling" attitude of responding to every serve.
10. Do anything to get the ball back. Be determined to meet the ball no matter how hard or where it is hit.

PROBLEM SOLVING

Problem	Probable Cause	Solution
Ball overpowers racket	Grip too loose	Hit the return with a vice-tight grip
Hitting too late	Slow racket preparation	Rotate upper body as soon as ball is sighted
	Too big of a backswing	Abbreviate backswing; keep racket behind ball
No pace on returned ball	Moving parallel with or diagonally away from baseline	Go to meet the ball; move diagonally forward

PROBLEM SOLVING

Problem	Probable Cause	Solution
No pace on returned ball	Listless racket	Thrust racket forward and downward through ball
Poor ball placement	No focusing intently on ball	See the ball twice: at impact on serve; refocus after bounce
	Not meeting ball early	Pick a spot before serve. Go meet the ball to hit it to that spot
Return goes too long	Not going forward; racket angled back	Meet ball early with squared-off racket face

ON THE COURT

A great way to sharpen your reflexes for service returns is to have your partner stand well inside their own baseline and bash serve after serve at you. Try to return each ball, whether it's in or not. Or play a game in which the receiver scores a point for each serve returned in-bounds. Or when your partner wants to hit a bucketful of practice serves, agree that you can also attempt returns on every ball.

On really hard serves to your backhand, try taking the ball with a two-handed return, even if you ordinarily hit a one-handed groundstroke. Using two hands helps to control the racket and keep it more stable, being better able to use the power already on the served ball. It also lets you take the ball a little earlier, which is essential if you want to be more aggressive on the return. In addition, if you're a bit late in getting the racket prepared, the other hand can help because you can make contact a little further back.

Gain some insight for knowing what kind of serve may be on its way by watching the ball toss, as follows:

- If the toss is high and forward, expect a flat serve.
- If the toss is low, expect a lollipop serve, so move in for an aggressive return.
- If the ball is tossed back over the server's head it will need spin to go in, so anticipate a topspin with its high kick-bounce.

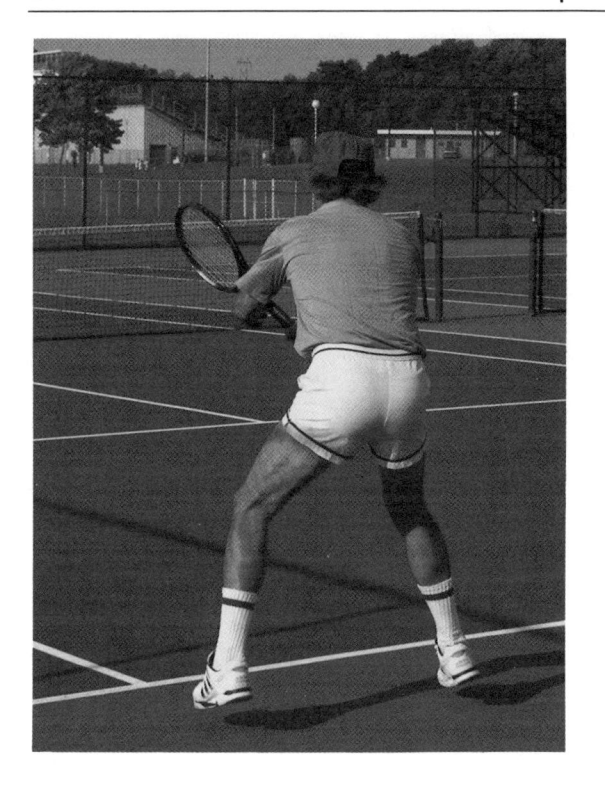

*Try a bouncing split-step as the ball is about to be served. This will give life to your whole body and responsiveness to your return. Make it a hopscotch kind of skip that energizes your legs and keeps your feet from being cemented to the court. Try to time the landing of your hop so that your feet hit the ground just as the server strikes the ball. Take the split-step slightly **forward** so you are ready to spring at the ball and use some linear momentum to hit the return.*

- If the ball is lifted to the outside, a slice is on the way, so the ball will stay low and bounce to the side.

Get into the habit of attacking the slower second serve. This will turn a defensive position into an offensive one and put enormous pressure on the server to get the first one in. Step in, take the ball on the rise, and drive a ground stroke deep and hard. Pick a target beforehand and try to hit that spot no matter where the serve goes

If you hit the ball well, continue your momentum to rush the net and take the weak reply early. It'll be a great psychological advantage in a match if you can take the net behind your own return.

Become good at returning serves. It will change the whole complexion of any match. If a big server knows you'll get the ball back, their pressure will rise with every return you hit. Let them know you're scrambling and not spectating.

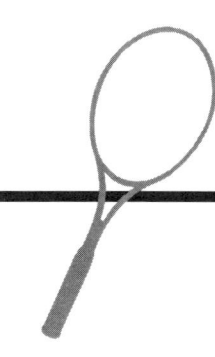

Chapter Five

Controlling the Forecourt

The liveliest tennis occurs at the net. It's arousing, vitalizing, invigorating, daring, reckless. It's the most adventurous part of the game.

Go into the forecourt often, for three reasons: (1) it provides a tactical advantage, (2) your presence alone can coerce mistakes from opponents, and (3) it adds dimension to the game. So pick up the tempo. Turn up the volume.

WHEN TO GO

Just be sure the moment is right. Everyone should carry a note taped to their racket that says: *caution — approach the net only under the following circumstances:*

1. **On a short ball.** If your opponent offers a shallow ball, that's in invitation to the forecourt. The further in front of the baseline you can move to hit, the more automatic your response should be to follow your shot to the net.
2. **Behind your own strong shot.** Go up to the net only when you hit a ball that you believe will force your opponent to reply with a lessened return. Usually this will be when you have your rival on the run or

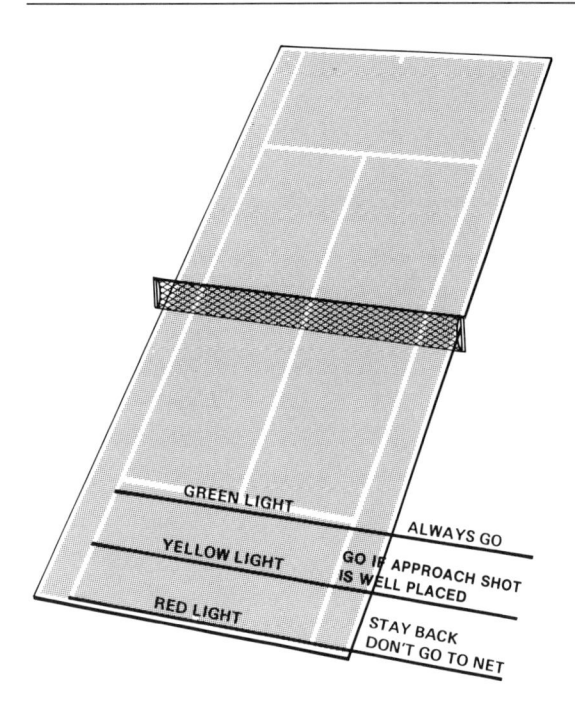

The baseline is a guide. When hitting from behind it, stay back, but the further in front of the baseline you can move to hit, the more inviting the net becomes.

otherwise off-balance, or when you've rifled a shot to their weaker side. There are other times when you simply "sense" that your shot will be overpowering enough to extract a feeble return.

HOW TO GET THERE

When you decide to take the net, commit your mind firmly to that intent, but make sure that you execute the complete approach shot first. Let the following guidelines govern your trip:

1. **Hit the approach shot deep.** A cardinal sin of tennis is to approach the net behind a ball hit too shallow in your opponent's court. It makes you vulnerable, giving too many options to your rival. The approach shot must put your opponent on the defensive, so send the ball deep, preferably to the weaker side.

2. **Sacrifice pace for placement.** Try for a winner if you have a wide open court, but be cautious not to overhit the approach shot. Take a shorter backswing, stroke through the ball, and hit for depth rather than speed. Make a definite follow-through in the direction of your target area.

3. **Hit the ball at the top of its bounce.** Move in to catch the ball high, where you'll have more margin of safety for net clearance. You'll also be closer to the net, and your opponent will have a little less time to respond. Take short stutter-steps as you approach the ball. Be sure to get your shoulders turned for the hit. Then keep moving forward as you make contact — not on a full running stride, but with a follow-through that allows you to transfer your weight into a continuation of your approach to the net.

4. **Follow the path of your shot.** Wherever you hit the ball, go directly behind it, on-line with its flight path. This will keep you in the middle of the widest area of possible return from your opponent.

5. **Split-step as your opponent is about to hit.** No matter where you are on the court, just as your rival is about to hit the ball, pull up to a controlled pause in your approach. Do a split-step to check your

A well-executed approach to the net will produce effective results. Hit the shot deep, stay on-line directly behind the path of your shot, pull up with a split-step as your opponent is about to hit, then finish the point off quickly.

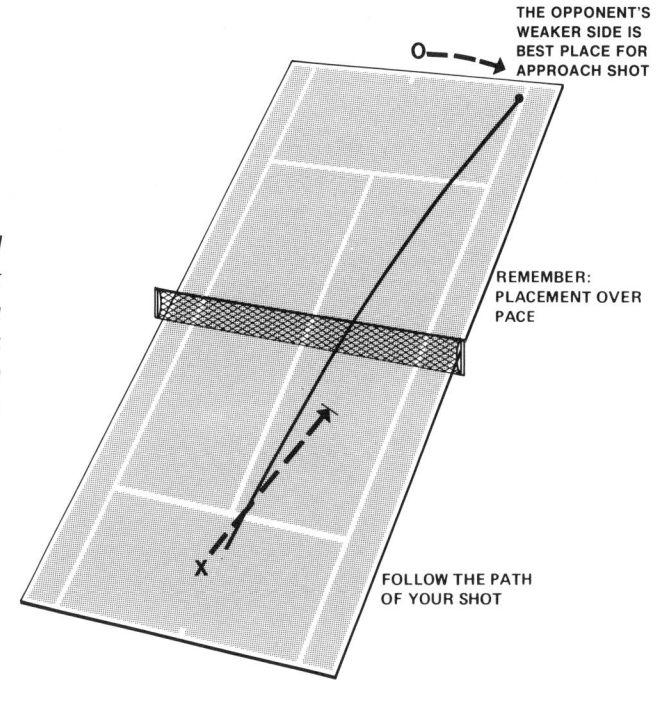

THE OPPONENT'S WEAKER SIDE IS BEST PLACE FOR APPROACH SHOT

REMEMBER: PLACEMENT OVER PACE

FOLLOW THE PATH OF YOUR SHOT

forward momentum. Hopscotch yourself into being ready to move in any direction, including backward if your opponent replies with a lob.

6. **Finish the point quickly.** Complete your trip to the net and become an aggressive opportunist. Have a finishing instinct. Win the point as quickly as you can.

Be selective about going to the net behind your serve. The best time is on a serve hit into the far corner of the advantage court, where it will pull the receiver off the court and also compel a weaker return (assuming the receiver is right-handed). Be cautious about following serves hit to a strong receiver's forehand side in the deuce court, for that presents the receiver with better angle possibilities for returning the ball past you.

AT THE NET

Tennis becomes condensed at the net, for the mechanical story of the volley stroke is brief:

1. The volley is a short stroke. It's a compact and firm block of the ball — a punch rather than a swing. Keep the racket solid with an asbestos hand.
2. The ball should be played early, before it gets to your side.

Whenever you can, hit a **drive** volley. Lengthen the swing, take the racket back a bit further, and give the stroke extra forward impulse. Instead of merely blocking the ball, **drill** it! Make the ball do something more than just using your strings as a trampoline.

Remember that you've come up to the net to win the point quickly. So drive the ball

Tennis for Experienced Players

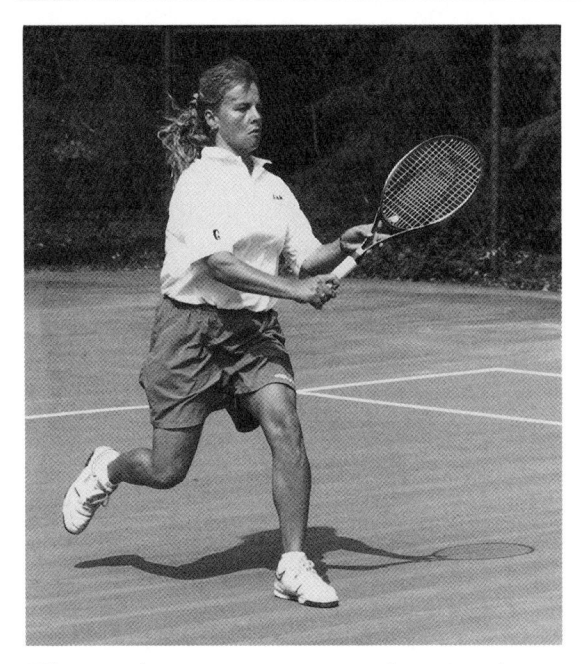

When you're on your way up to the net and your opponent is about to strike a return . . .

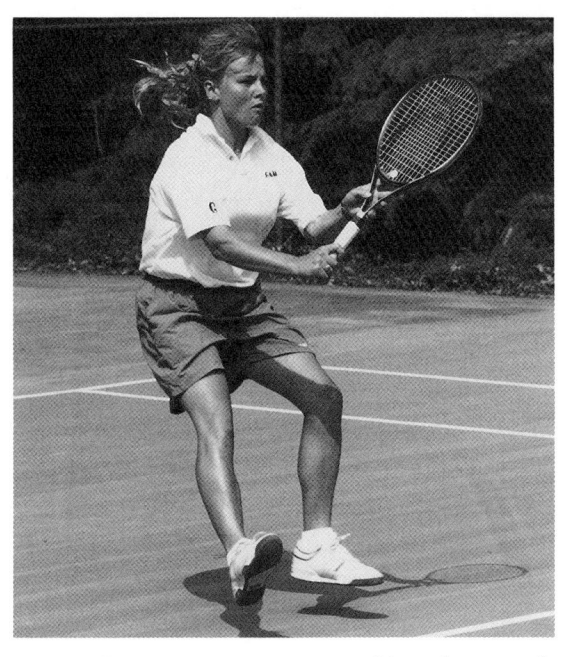

. . . collect your momentum with a hopscotch split-step into a ready-to-react position . . .

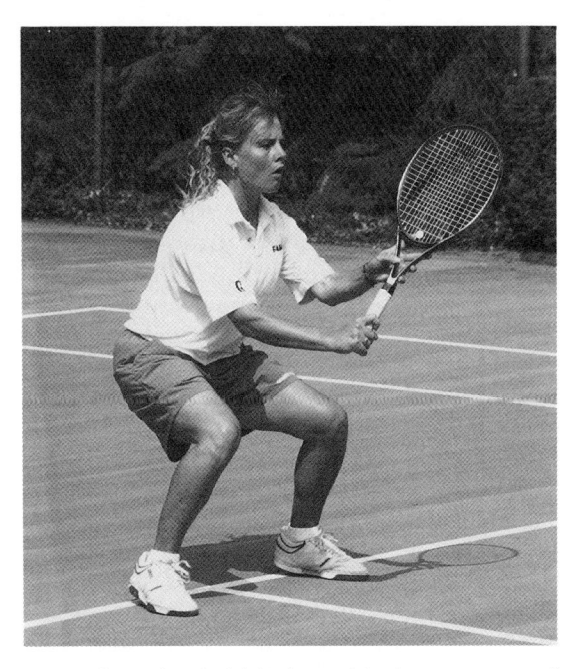

. . with racket held high and in front, prepared for a quick response in any direction.

out of your opponent's reach. Hit it with an attitude of: "**there** — take **that!**"

Try hitting down on the ball, just like when you're giving backspin to a driving groundstroke. Thrust the racket into and down the back of the ball. Not with a karate chop, but rather **through** the ball. This will add strength to your stroke and pace to the resulting shot.

If you have pushed your opponent off to one side of the court, drift to that side. The further off the court your rival is, the more you can forget about protecting against a shot coming behind you, since few players can take a wide ball and spin it cross-court with the angle it would need to stay in-bounds.

When forced wide for your own volley stroke, you generally have two choices for

Controlling the Forecourt

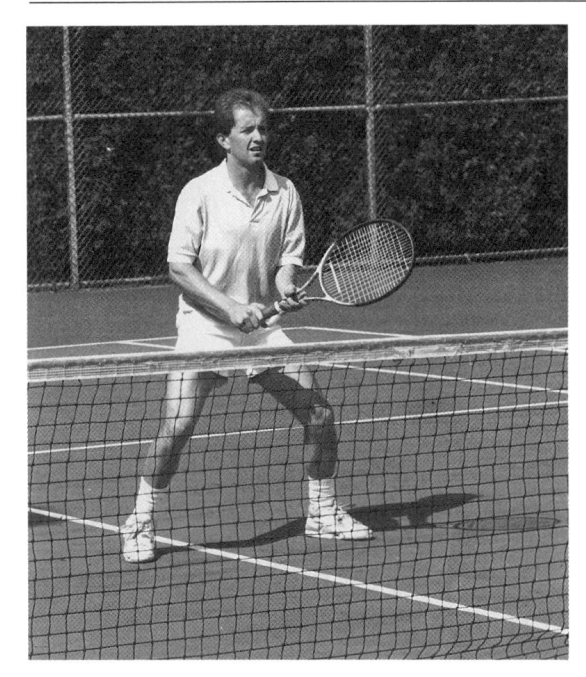

There's nothing elaborate about a volley. Just be ready to attack the ball . . .

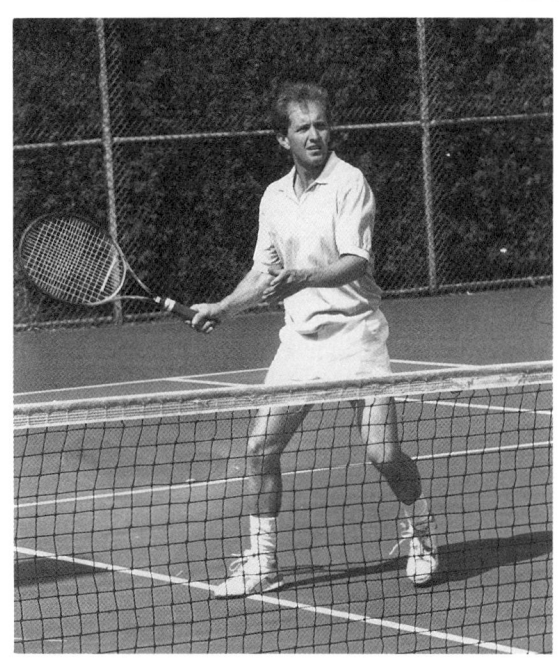

. . . then take a short backswing, keeping the grip firm . . .

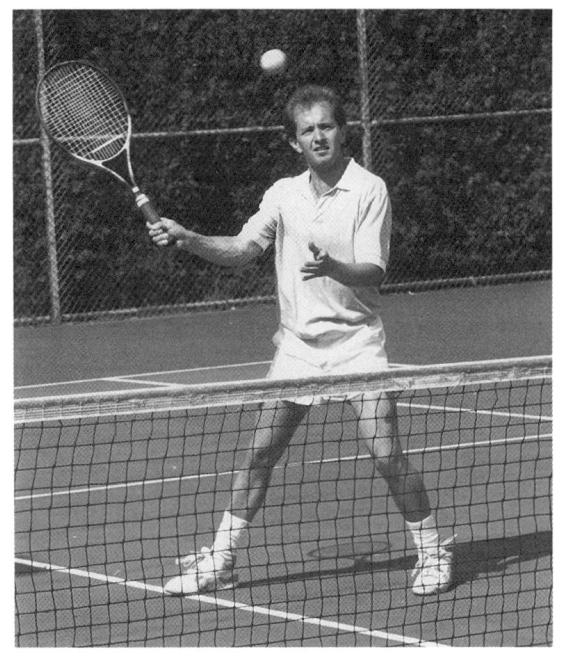

. . . and smack the racket affirmatively into the ball, making contact early . . .

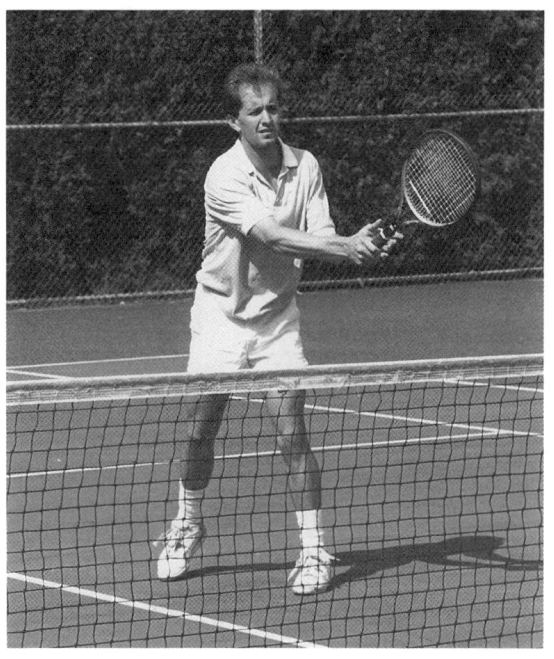

. . . to punch it away from your opponent and win the point right away.

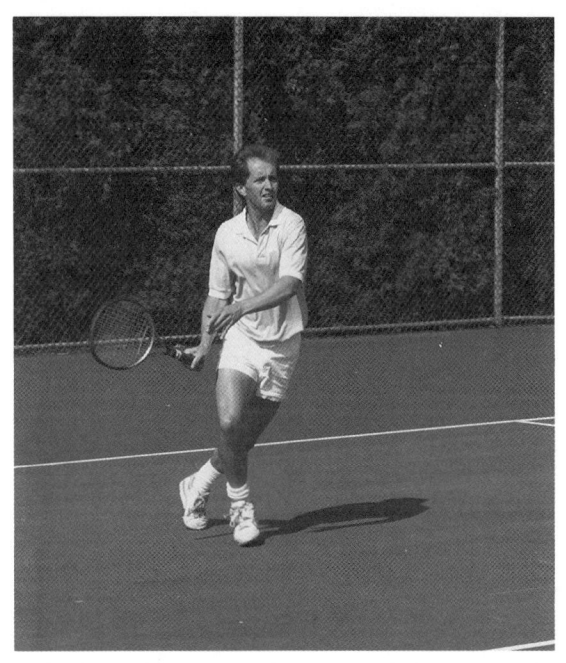

When you have enough time, and the approaching ball is not overpowering . . .

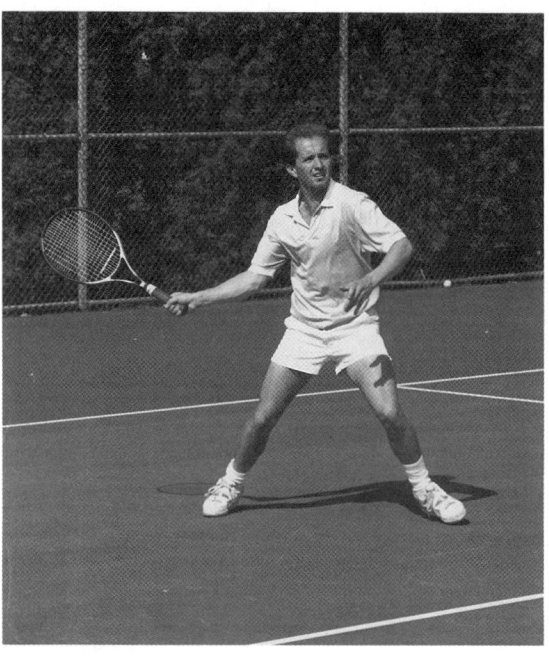

. . . step up to hit a drive volley. Take a longer backswing, and . . .

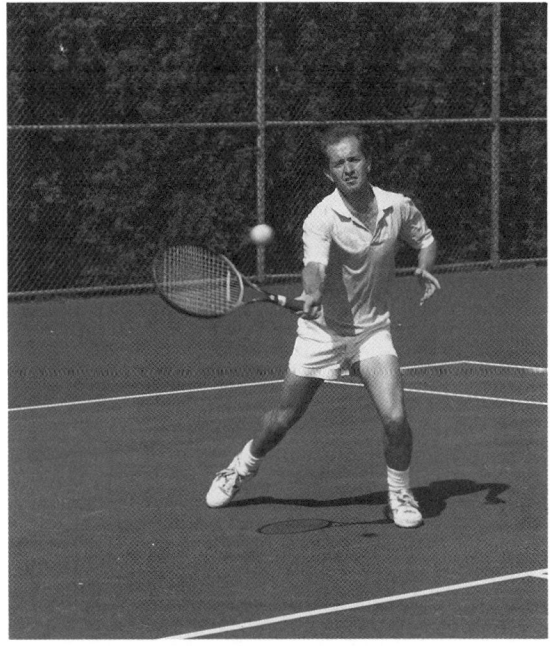

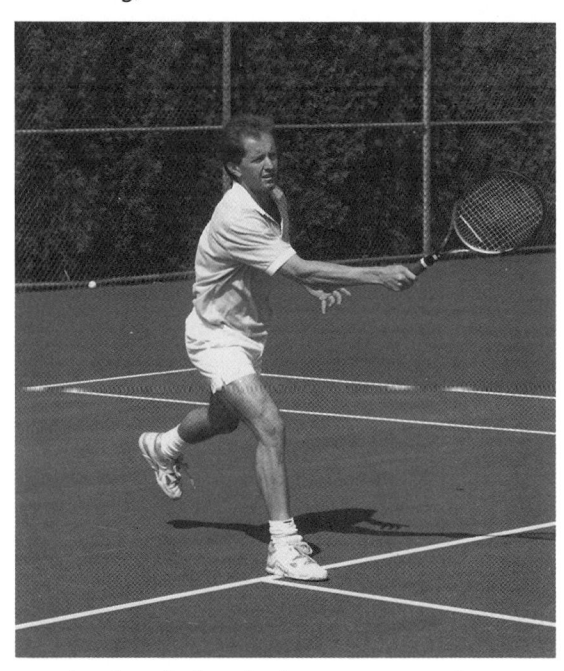

. . . drill the racket convincingly into the ball . . .

. . . to place it deep in the court, away from your opponent.

ball placement: a drive volley hit down the line as deep as possible, or a sharply angled cross-court shot. The cross-court option may be safer, especially when the ball comes low to you. Give the ball enough lift for ample net clearance, and you'll find that the severe angle you can give to this shot will keep it out of the range of any opponent. A down-the-line volley leaves less room for error, but there are times when such a placement, if hit affirmatively and deep enough, can "wrong-foot" an opponent who is on the move anticipating a cross-court volley.

REMINDERS

1. Go up to the net only when you can hit from in front of the baseline (the serve is an exception).
2. Hit the approach shot deep, preferably to the opponent's weaker side.
3. Come to a split-step pause as your opponent is about to hit, weight still in controlled momentum.
4. Hit a drive volley for a winner or, otherwise at least place the next ball deep.
5. Win the point as quickly as you can.
6. Try to hit every volley out of reach of your opponent.
7. The best placements are deep down-the-line, or shallow cross-court.
8. Be aggressive at the net. Attack the ball. Defend the net like a hockey goalie.

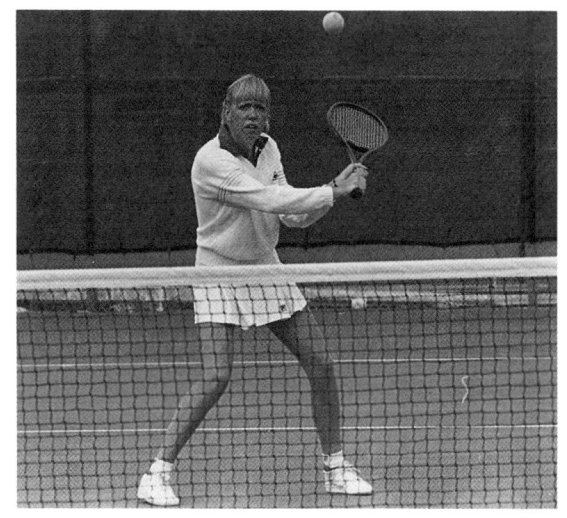

To give stability to a volley stroke and pace to the shot, tilt the racket head back slightly and . . .

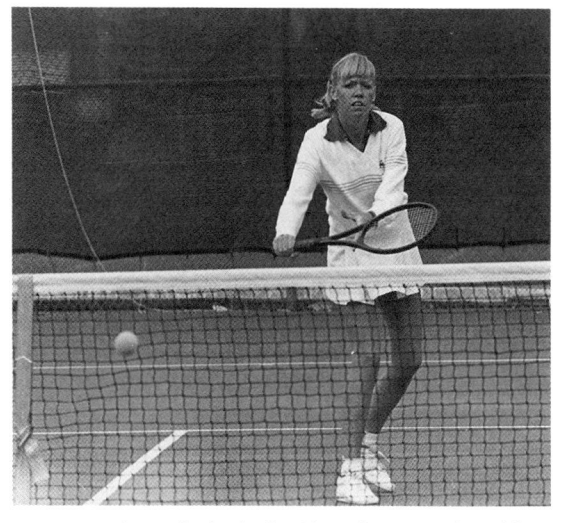

. . . come through the ball with a downward and forward thrust, keeping a steady wrist for the contact.

PROBLEM SOLVING

Problem	Probable Cause	Solution
Getting passed on the way up to the net	Approach shot hit too shallow	Use more follow-through to hit approach shot deep to weaker side
Late ball contact	Not pausing on approach	Split-step into controlled pause as return is about to be hit
	Arms held too tight to body in volley position	Hold elbows away from body; keep racket head up
	Too much of a backswing	Keep swing compact, with minimal take-back of racket
No strength to stroke	Racket head getting ahead of hand	Keep forearm behind racket on forehand; parallel to racket on backhand
	Grip not firm	Squeeze racket tight just before contact
	Racket head quitting	Punch crisply down and through the back of the ball
Trouble controlling ball placement	Defensive attitude at net	Attack the ball; hit early in flight
	Indecisiveness	Pick a spot away from opponent; rifle ball into that spot

Controlling the Forecourt 67

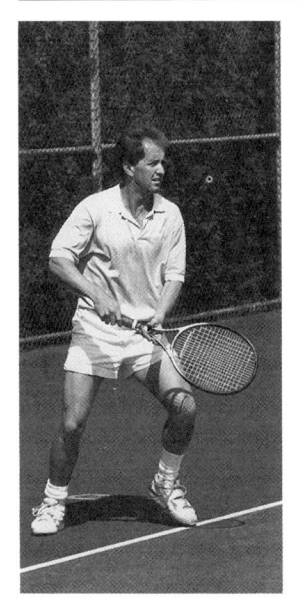

When you must lunge for a wide ball, take a short "jab" step with your lead foot . . .

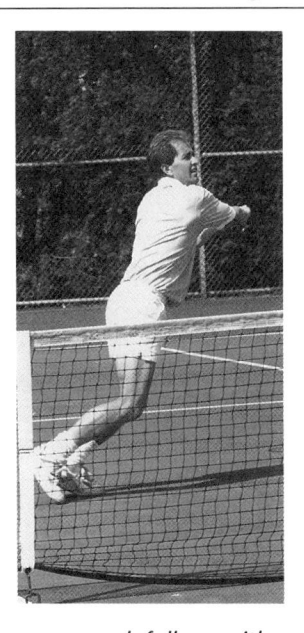

. . . and follow with a cross-over step with your trail foot . . .

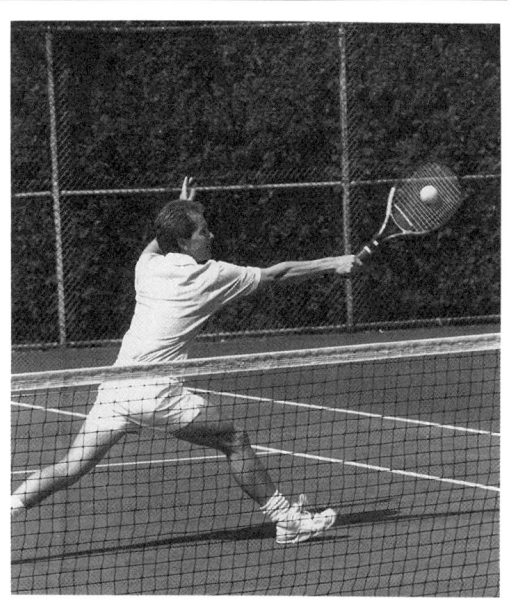

. . . for a two-step maneuver which should get you quickly in range to return the ball.

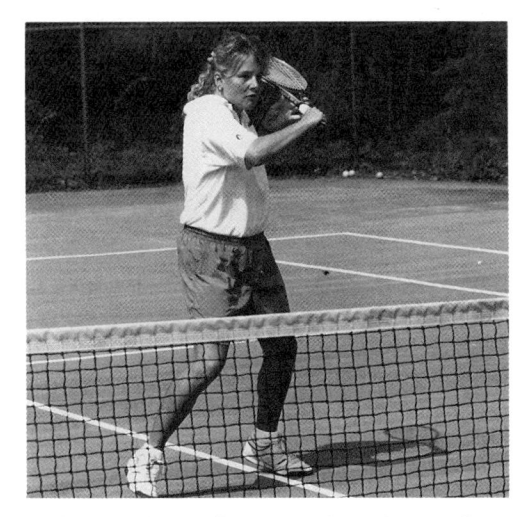

When you're well stationed at the net for a volley, and your opponent sends a bullet right at you . . .

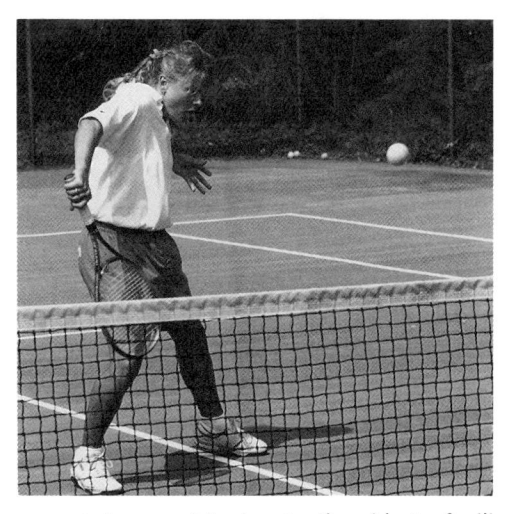

. . . take a quick step to the side to facilitate a brief shoulder turn and get your upper body away from the ball. Keep a vice-tight grip; block the ball back as best you can.

OVERHEADS

When you're at the net and you see your opponent:

- leaning back,
- taking a short backswing, or
- tilting the racket face back,

you can expect a lob. Start backpedaling in anticipation.

If the lob is too short, let fly with an overhead. Hit it for a winner. Give it an air of finality. It'll provide you with a sense of vibrance that will permeate the rest of your game.

The overhead is often likened to a serve — with added choreography. Except that:

1. The ball isn't where you want it. You must get **in back** of the ball. Shuffle-step into position. Keep your legs alive, with knees bent, for last-minute adjustments.
2. The windup is more compact. Forget any fancy takeback of the racket. Just get it up over your shoulder like you were an archer reaching back to pull an arrow out of the quiver. Use your serving grip, but hit the ball flat, without topspin.

As you shuffle into position, **sharpen your focus on the ball.** Bring your weight to your

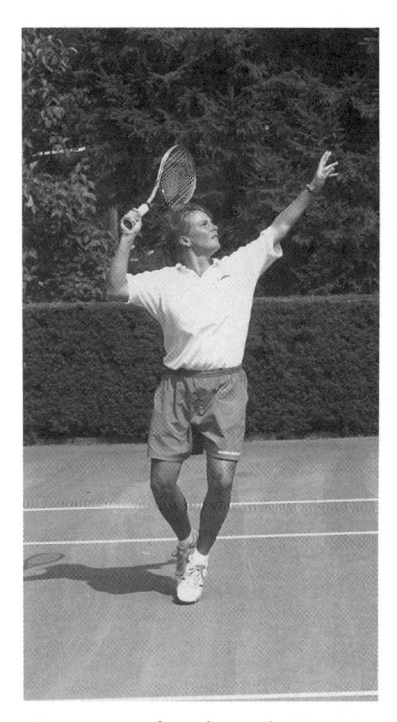

For an overhead, get behind the ball. Pull shoulders well around. Focus intently on the ball.

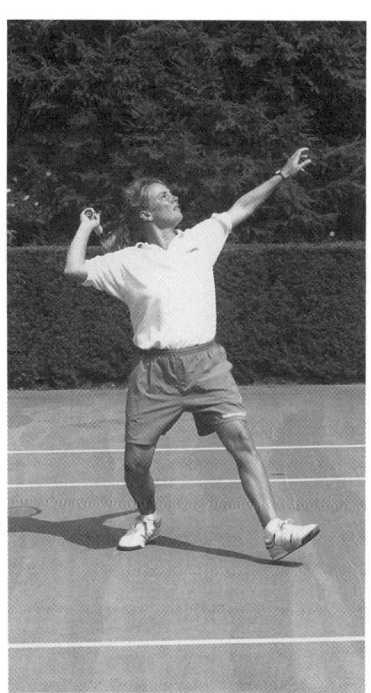

Bring the racket back as for a serve, only with less windup. Keep the backswing simple.

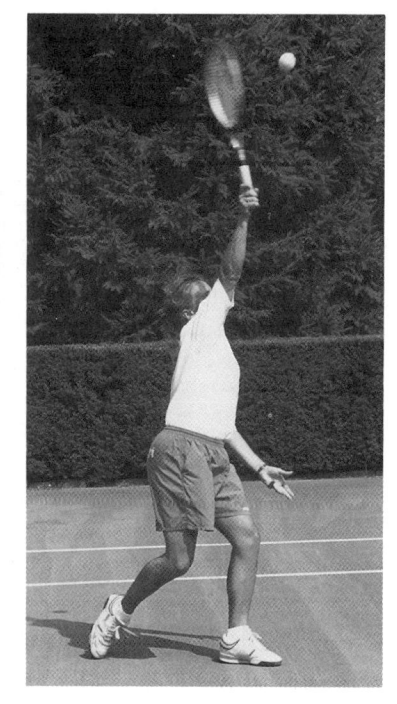

Make contact more in front than for a serve. Hit the ball with as much power as you can control.

back foot as you prepare the racket. Get your shoulders well turned, ninety degrees to the net.

Contrary to what you may have been led to believe, it is not mandatory to hit full throttle on every overhead. Spank the ball with only as much effort as you can handle, and place it deep to remain in control of the point.

But when you can, go for a winner. The older name for this shot is a smash — a descriptive term that told what to do with the ball. So crack off a big shot — **smash it!**

REMINDERS

1. Get into position early. It's better to be too far behind the ball than too far under it.
2. Keep life in your legs for final adjustments.
3. Bring the racket straight back; nothing fancy. But get a good shoulder rotation.
4. Watch the ball intently, perhaps lifting your nonhitting hand (or elbow) up toward the ball to track its flight.
5. Hit the ball flat; no attempted spin.
6. Hit it with as much power as you can while still having control of the placement.
7. Extend into the ball with a full pendular swing; no hunched-shoulder attempts.

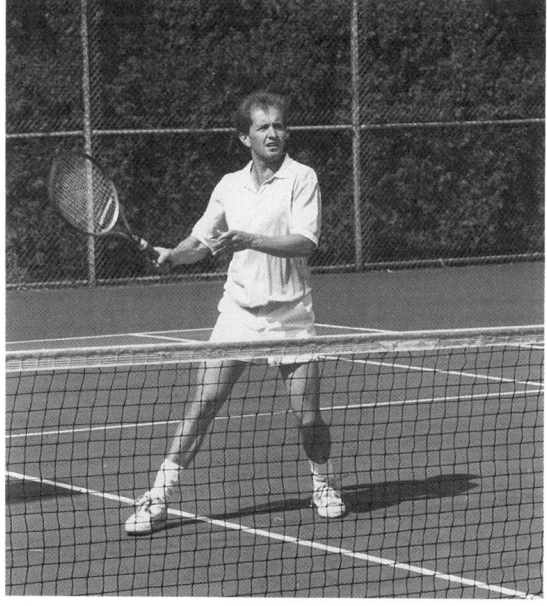

There is often a moment — when a ball comes high to your forehand — that forces a quick decision: should you smash it or hit a volley stroke?

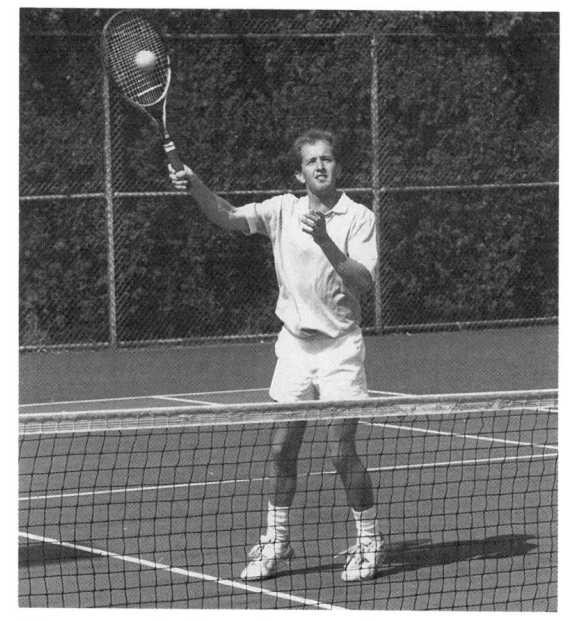

The answer is direct: if you can't get your arm up and extended for a free-wheeling overhead, then volley the ball. Be sure to keep your arm extra firm for this high stroke.

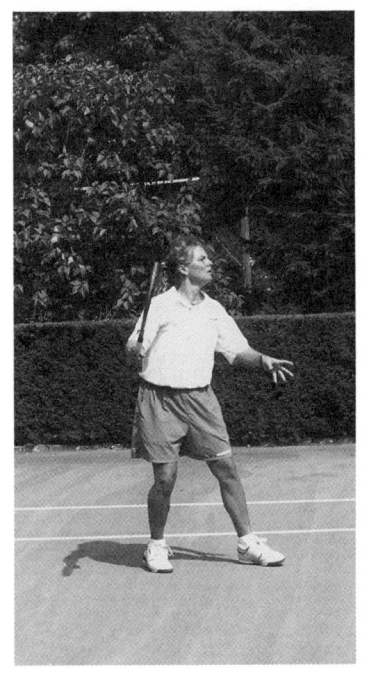

Here's a vibrant skill used to intercept a lob that would otherwise land behind you. Do a quick retreat of shuffle steps, get your shoulders turned well around, then . . .

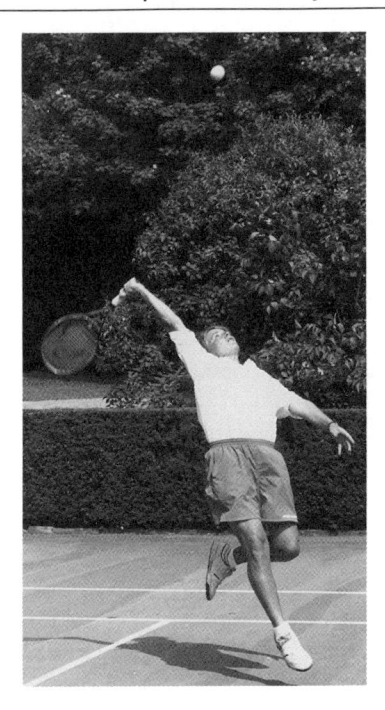

. . . lunge into a jump overhead. Spring off your feet. Give plenty of whip to your arm and especially your wrist to get the racket up and forward for the late contact point.

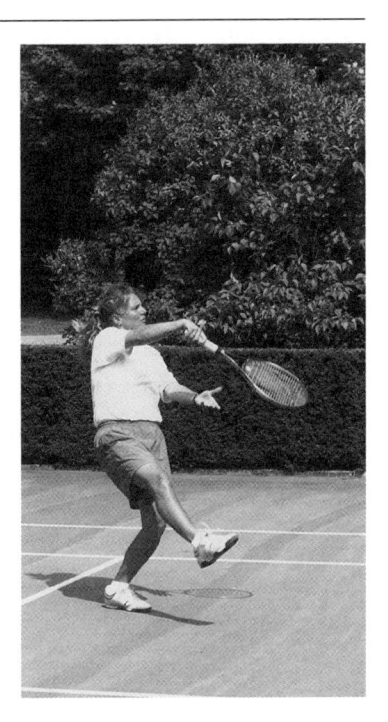

Finish off the stroke. It's common to be conservative on a jump overhead. Instead, hit the ball with explosive flair. Lash your body upward — your arm and wrist forward.

PROBLEM SOLVING

Problem	Probable Cause	Solution
Ball hit into net	Trying to hit too hard	Swing only as hard as you can control
	Pulling head down just before contact	Keep chin up until after contact
	Letting ball drop too far	Hit at full extension of arm
	Throwing hips back into jackknife during hit	Hit with forward-shifting weight, as in serve
Ball hit too long	Contact point too far back	Set well up behind ball
	Elbow leading swing, racket trailing at contact	Use serve-like fling of racket, arm extending through swing
	Punching at ball	Use fluid, pendular swing; not a push
	Sidearm swing	Get elbow up; bring racket up and over

ON THE COURT

It's part mind-game, playing at the net. If you still do not have a point-finishing instinct, spend a good portion of every practice session in the forecourt.

Even rehearse some shots while stationed in that awkward position on the court euphemistically called "no-man's land" (at mid-court, near the service line). Learn that you can move in to the ball and knock off drive volleys, keeping them deep and low, for outright winners or to improve your court position.

Should you change grip, forehand and backhand, for the volley? Sometimes a Continental grip is suggested for both sides, its advantage being that it's a time-saver and its natural backward tilt of the racket on both sides works in favor of a stabilizing downward smack at the ball. However, there is a tendency for the racket to be too severely angled on the backhand. Furthermore, analysis of the pro players reveals that there is almost always some degree of hand shift from side to side. The change is not as dramatic as for a ground stroke, but enough to get a more effective racket angle at impact. Most often, they hit with a Continental grip on the forehand side and a slight shift toward the top of the handle for a backhand. In most cases, for players of all levels, there is ample time to make this shift.

An energizing volley drill, which will help you with switching grips, is for you and your partner to stand across the net from one another, each in the forecourt. Keep a ball alive, hitting firmly but within each other's reach. Play volley against volley, trying to hit as many consecutive shots as the two of you can manage.

Another excellent practice drill is to divide the court in half longitudinally, so that only half the court, with the service area and the backcourt behind it, is considered in bounds. A point is scored by any ball that lands behind the service line and inside the baseline. Take up volleying positions just behind the service line, bounce the ball to start a rally, and attempt to drive the ball past your partner.

In any volley drill, get in the habit of making an immediate shoulder turn sideways as soon as the ball leaves the other player's racket. This will coil your body for a stinging volley, and it sets you up to push off quickly to reach a ball wide to your side. If you keep your swing compact, this shoulder turn will make solid contact with the ball fairly easy.

Don't ignore practicing the timing of the split-step as you approach the net. Land into this ready-to-respond position **just as the opponent makes contact with the ball.** Create a slight imbalance forward in your split-step, then bounce out of it by picking up your forward momentum again to go at the ball.

Ask your practice partner to lift up some really high lobs. Know where the threshold is — at what point is the ball too high to be effectively smashed from flight, and when should it be allowed to bounce? If you let it bounce, you'll find that you can add some spin to your overhead, much like a topspin serve, to arc the ball into the court.

Learn how flat-out you can swing with your overhead and still control the destiny of the ball. Become accustomed to hitting with unrestricted conviction. Soon you'll be elated after every overhead instead of agonized.

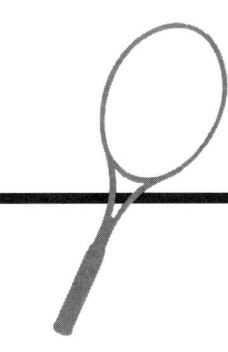

Chapter Six

Hitting Point-Winning Lobs

The poor lob. It's the orphan of tennis — a devalued shot that is often ignored, much unused. But it can:

- buy you time when you need to recover court position.
- dislodge an aggressive forecourt player away from the net.
- drag down a strong hitter with its change of pace.
- be hit for an outright winner.

The lob provides one of the game's most satisfying moments — when you loft a ball just over a net player's reach and watch that player's hopeless effort of trying to chase it down. To hit such a shot is a sign of a finished player.

TWO KINDS OF LOBS

The lob has two variations, each with its own purpose. An **offensive lob** is hit against a player at the net, lifted just over that player's reach to land in the backcourt where it should outrun any attempt at a retrieval. Thus it's hit as a concluding shot, with the anticipation of it being a point winner.

On the other hand, a **defensive lob** is hit as self-preservation by keeping the ball in play to salvage staying in a point. The most common use is when an opponent has driven you off the side of the court, and you need time to get back. It can also be hit whenever your rival has pressed you into an awkward off-balance predicament that keeps you from

Tennis for Experienced Players

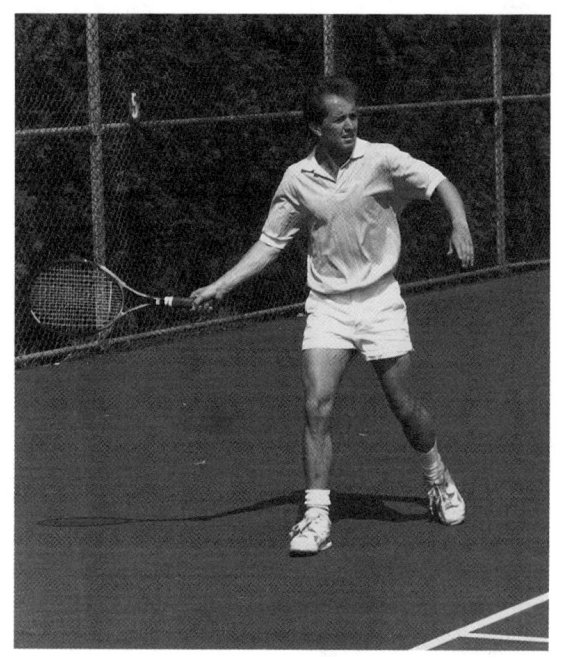

An offensive lob is a compact groundstroke, with a low backswing so that . . .

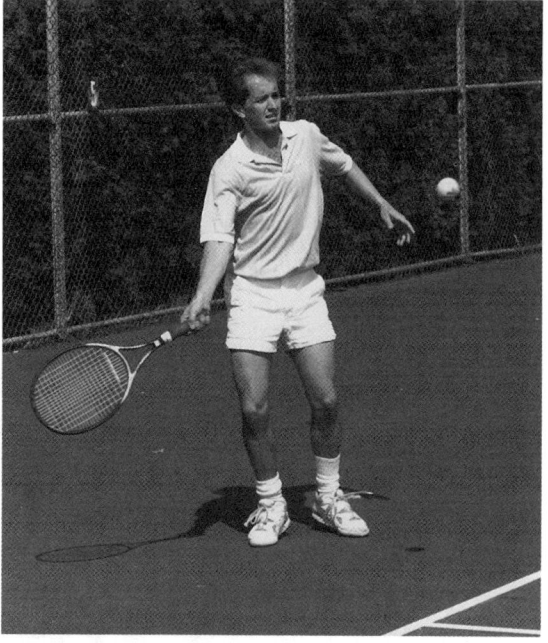

. . . the racket can be brought into the ball from below the point of contact, wrist held steady . . .

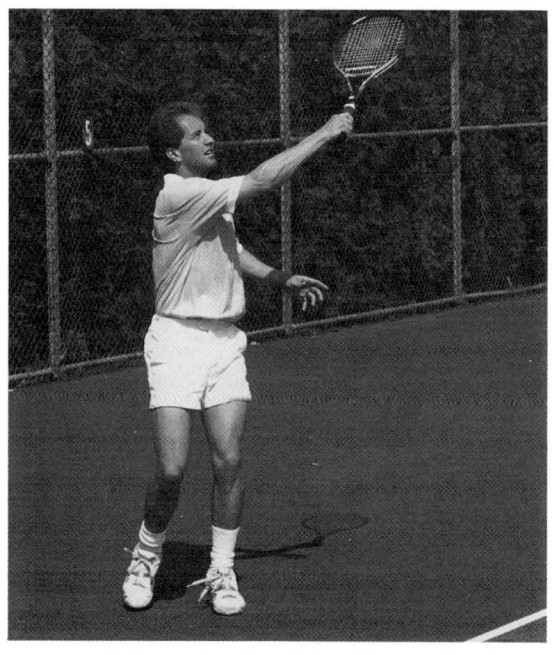

. . . and the racket head completing the stroke by following the trajectory of the ball.

hitting a strong shot. Thus, a defensive lob is hit higher, its virtue being to allow you to recollect yourself for the next shot.

HIT OFFENSIVE LOBS FOR WINNERS

An offensive lob is needed when your rival has taken up a station at the net. Lift the ball so that the highest point of its travel is just a couple of feet higher than your opponent can reach.

There's no need to change the grip, for the lob is essentially a groundstroke lifted high. Make your swing more compact, shorten the backswing and take the racket back lower than the point of contact. Tilt the racket face back to align it for the upward hit.

Come into the ball from below the point of contact, low to high, then spank the ball with the strings held steady at **exactly ninety degrees to the intended trajectory of the shot.** Let the racket head follow-through into the lofted path of the airborne ball — no higher. Hit it softly, delicately. Lay the ball on an imaginary cloud above your opponent.

Relax your hitting elbow as you bring the racket forward, but keep the wrist steady to avoid the tendency of giving an extra flick of the wrist in a subconscious effort to lift the ball. Bend your knees more than for a groundstroke as you prepare for the hit, then unbend them with your swing to help add to the incline direction of the racket. On the backhand side, which is considerably more difficult for most players, emphasize the upward follow-through of the racket head, and give the ball a little extra room for error by lifting it higher than on a forehand lob.

GIVE DEFENSIVE LOBS HEIGHT

You desperately need a defensive lob when your opponent has dragged you off the side of the court and has come up to the net ready to pounce on a low return. And the more you're pressed into hitting on the run, the less likely it is that you'll be able to get off a fully controlled, offensive shot. So drop the racket head down extra low; tilt the face back, and let fly with a limber-arm upward swing. Do whatever you can to get the ball back **high**. Use the shot to push your opponent away from the net and to give yourself time to recover your court position. Don't be conservative with defensive lobs. Lift the ball into the stratosphere. Give yourself enough time to retie your shoelaces and still get back to the court.

SPIN FOR THE LOB

A topspin lob is one of the joyful sights of tennis. The ball arches just over a flabbergasted net player, then bends into the court and kicks toward the fence. Properly hit, it's a sure point-winner.

To give topspin to a lob, you must get the racket head especially low to start. Let your elbow relax and lay your wrist back, then release a vigorous upward flail of your arm, without losing control. Finish high above your opposite shoulder. Fling the racket like you were going to throw it into the ozone layer. Use lots of wrist.

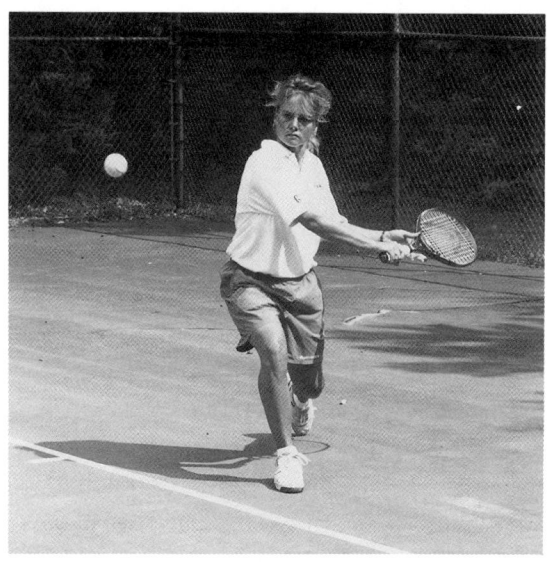

A backhand lob is usually more challenging, so make sure the racket head drops low in the backswing . . .

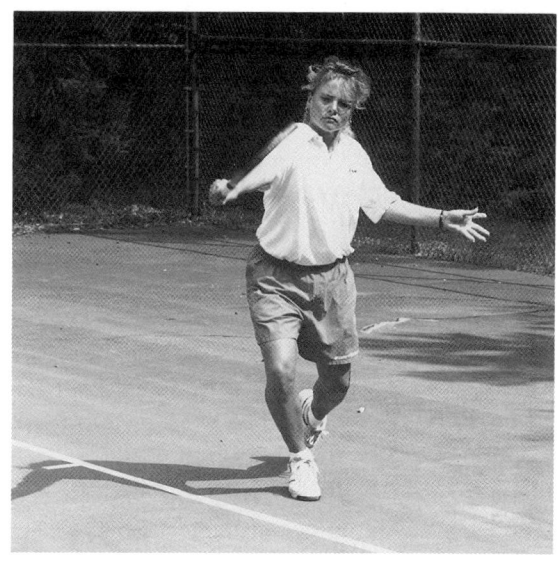

. . . for its upward path into the ball. Keep the wrist positively steady for the hit, then . . .

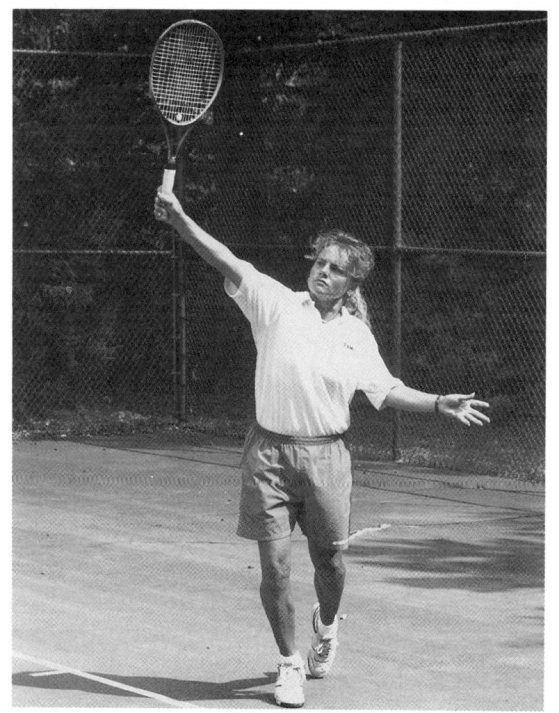

. . . emphasize the height of the follow-through to give more lift to the ball for an extra allowance for error.

A topspin lob is difficult to produce on the backhand side. Furthermore, it cannot be hit from a contact point below the waist, and is difficult to control when the oncoming ball has good pace.

By contrast, a backspin lob is a fine advantage when under extreme pressure from a well-paced ball or when forced off the side of the court. In its flight the ball will float, then fall to rebound passively. Its lazy path takes the psychological advantage from an aggressive net-player and gives you extra time to recollect yourself for the continuation of the point.

Start the racket higher for this shot, then push the racket into the ball with its face laid back. The swing should be essentially parallel with the court. Deflect the ball into generous height, and always aim to land in the backcourt.

Hitting Point-Winning Lobs

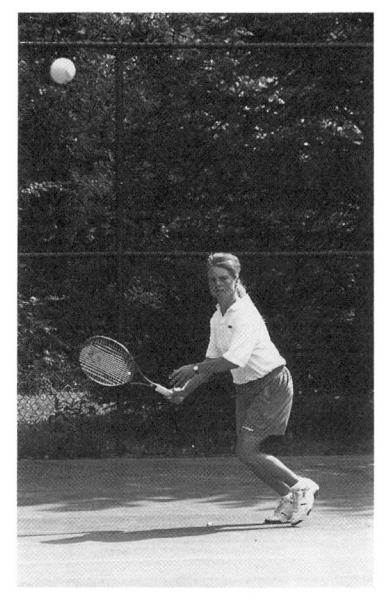

When your opponent has pushed you off the side of the court and has an established net position . . .

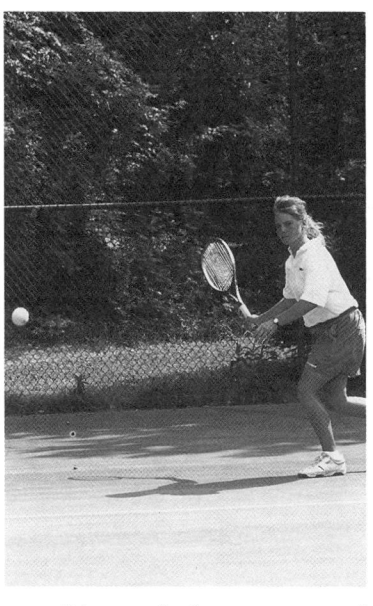

. . . it's usually best to respond with a defensive lob . . .

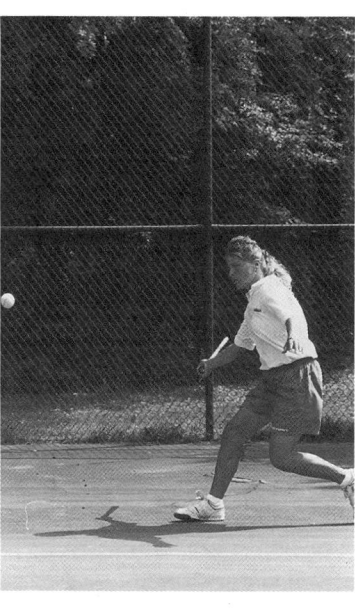

. . . whereby you need to drop the racket head down extra low . . .

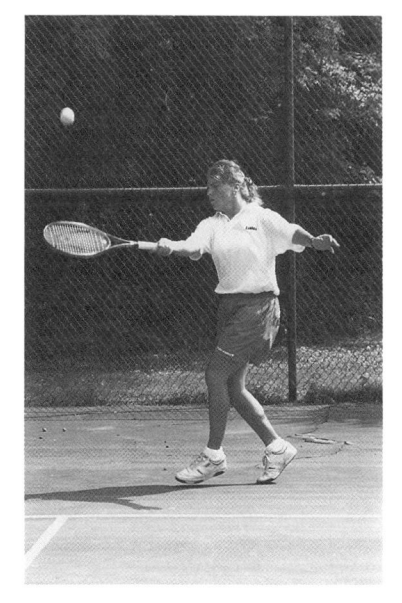

. . . and come up under the ball with a loose-arm swing . . .

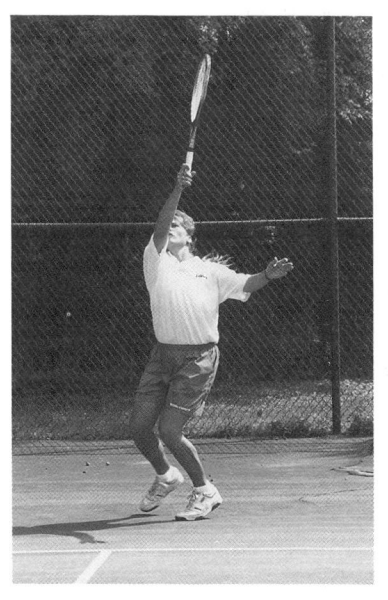

. . . that will give the ball plenty of height and provide you with enough time . . .

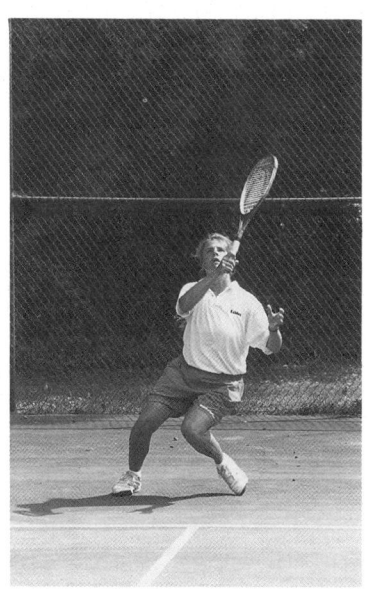

. . . to slam on the brakes and scramble back to your court position.

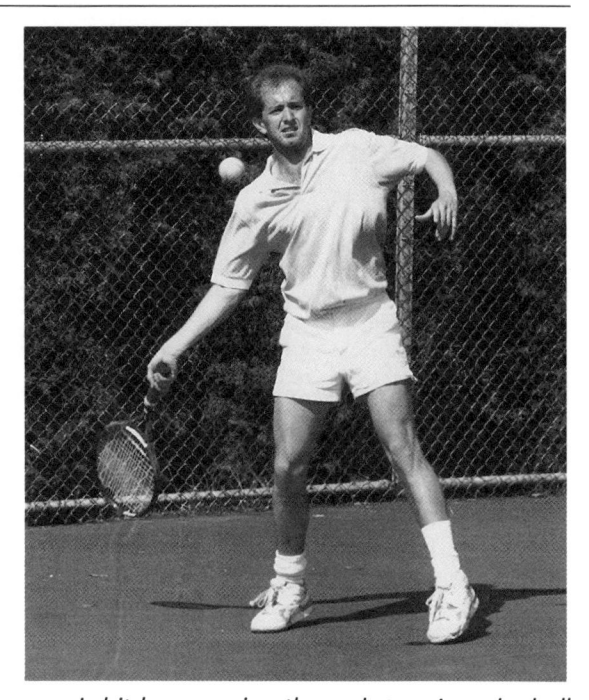

The topspin lob is a flamboyant, freewheeling swat of the ball which . . .

. . . is hit by sweeping the racket up into the ball from several feet below the contact point . . .

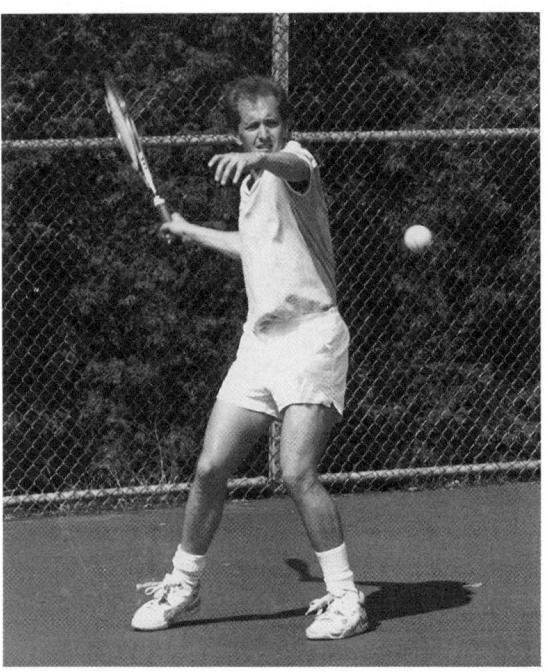

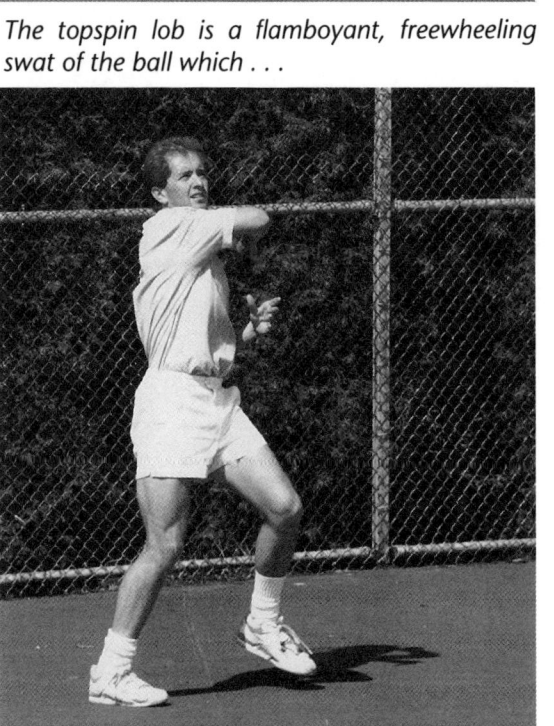

. . . with a vigorous upward fling of the arm and wrist to finish high across the opposite shoulder.

USING LOBS IN MATCH PLAY

Don't keep the lob in reserve just for use against a net player. Hit it whenever you are pinned into a defensive position and need time for recovery, or as a change of pace against a strong hitter, or simply to break up the rhythm of a prolonged rally.

If the sun is behind one end of the court, use a lob often when it will force your opponent to look up into it. But don't lift a lob up with a wind that is coming from behind you. Hit it into the wind instead, with extra impulse so it still lands deep.

When pushed off the side of the court, angle the lob cross-court, where there's more hitting room. Otherwise, hit the lob over the backhand side of a net player where, if it falls short of enough height, it will at least force an awkward high backhand from your rival.

Anytime you hit an offensive lob over a net player, your first impulse should be to follow it to the net. Even if your opponent manages to chase the ball down, the return will have diluted strength. Often, your foe will toss up another lob of their own in desperation. Either way, it will be opportune for you to be in the forecourt to volley away the weakened reply.

In every match, try a few lobs early, even if your opponent does not come to the net. There is a tendency in a match to hit the first few lobs too short, probably because the muscles are still tight. By lofting a couple of high shots early in the match, you'll get your bearings set for the first time you need it to go over your opponent's head.

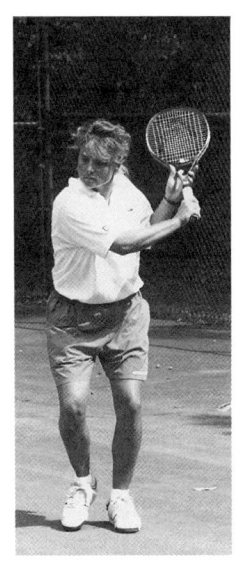

To give backspin to a lob the racket should be brought back higher . . .

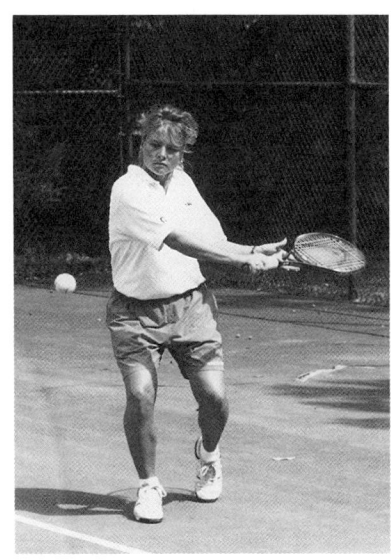

. . . then forward into the ball on an essentially level plane . . .

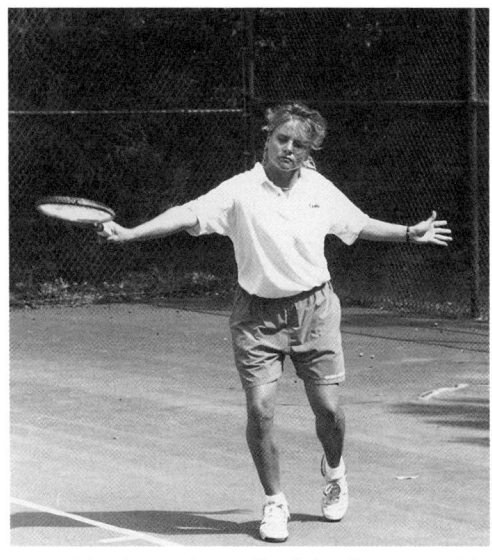

. . with the strings tilted back to provide spin and plenty of loft.

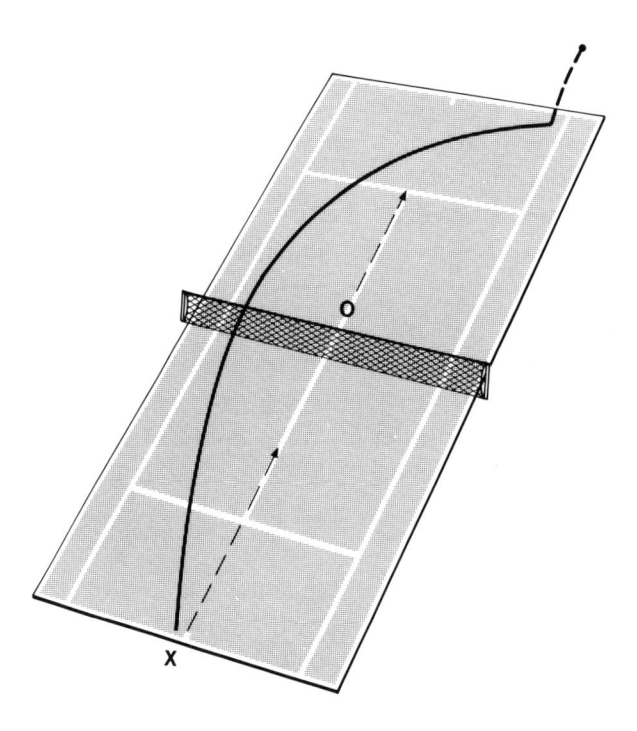

When you deliver a well-hit offensive lob, particularly if it's placed to the backhand side of your opponent, you should follow the shot by going quickly up to the net to volley away the anticipated weak return.

REMINDERS

1. Hit the lob as an offensive shot whenever you can. Try to win the point directly.
2. Hit defensive lobs when necessary. Give them plenty of height.
3. Always provide enough clearance — hit too high rather than too low.
4. Swing the racket directly up in the same plane as the height you want to give to the ball, and follow through into that trajectory.
5. Have the strings flattened against the intended height of the shot at contact.
6. Keep a steady wrist for lobs hit without spin, but give the arm and wrist lots of whip for topspin lobs.
7. When under pressure, do anything to get the ball back high and deep.

PROBLEM SOLVING

Problem	Probable Cause	Solution
Erratic control	Stopping racket too soon	Hit through the ball, racket following intended path
Hitting too short	Racket head not dropped below point of contact	Get racket down; come up under ball
	Wrist too flaccid	Keep firm wrist throughout swing; aim for baseline
Hitting too long	Too big of a swing	Keep backswing short, but still follow through
	Flicking at ball with wrist	Keep wrist and forearm steady for swing
Not enough ball rotation on topspin lob	Conservative swing	Hit with whip-like swing of arm; plenty of wrist. Come emphatically up

ON THE COURT

When hitting lobs in match play, there is often an irresistible urge to keep a wary eye on your opponent — and this causes your arm to tighten. Practice the lob by trying a camera trick: focus on the ball and make the background fuzzy. You're still aware of the background, but it's out of focus, while the ball is a clear image.

Have your practice partner stand near the net, then bounce-hit a series of wide feeds to you on alternating sides, in rapid succession. In a match, as fatigue begins to have an effect, there is an increasing tendency to hit lobs too low. In this tiring practice you will learn how much more you'll need to lift the ball to have it accomplish its task.

When on the run to retrieve a wide shot, experiment with hitting an offensive lob, but only if you can steady yourself with a sound base to hit from. Give extra whip to your arm if you're still moving sidewards.

When your feeder is at the net while you practice lobs, have that partner smash every ball that you hit too short. Then get into the habit of trying to anticipate where the smash will go. In a match, it's too easy to concede the point when you see your lob fall short. But now, as you watch your partner crank up for an overhead, notice the shoulders and direction of the backswing — they will be aligned with the point of aim. Then scramble to that side. If you guess correctly in a match you may be able to lift up another lob, more deeply this time, and take the momentum away from your surprised adversary who had expected to end the point.

Occasionally, hit some lobs extra high. See how far into the clouds you can lift the ball while still keeping it in bounds. Then your regular-height defensive lobs will seem like a cinch.

It's the offensive lob, however, which often is ignored in practice sessions. Learn to desensitize yourself from the net player by pretending there is a ten-foot fence at the net. Think of the fence, not your opponent, as you hit shot after shot adroitly over the fence-net. Eventually your biggest problem will be to keep from laughing as you watch bewildered opponents try to retrieve the ball.

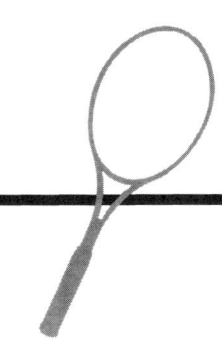

Chapter Seven

Making Extraordinary Shots Ordinary

In competition, you are compelled to hit running forehands, lunging overheads, half-volleys, double-jointed backhands, and other shots that seldom get practiced yet are part of every match you play. Tennis is a sport of constant motion, with microsecond changes of situation, and your success depends a great deal on your ability to adapt and hit from unconventional positions.

HITTING ON THE RUN

When having to chase down a wide shot and make a return while on the run, try the following:

1. **Cut the ball off early.** Just as for a return of serve, try to intercept the ball before it has moved too far off the court. Make a quick pivot, and go on a direct path ninety degrees to the line of flight of the ball. Cut it off early, before it gets out of your reach. As you approach the ball, stutter-step to gain the best hitting position, then try to give some linear momentum to your swing.
2. **Delay the backswing.** Never mind trying to get the racket back early. Pivot and run, using both arms in a pumping action to help your acceleration. Your first objective is to get to where you need to be. As you near the ball, abbreviate the backswing to

conserve time. Add a little loop to the forehand to help the timing and make the momentum of the swing continuous. Backhands may need some under-cutting.

3. **Let your arm propel the racket.** You may not be able to get your shoulders rotated in normal fashion, so you must rely on your arm to do most of the work. Keep your arm loose. Give it a whip that feels like the motion came from your shoulder socket, and add some flick of the wrist. Don't try to muscle the ball over the net, for this will only reduce the flinging action of the racket head and rob the swing of impulse.

4. **Provide an extra margin of safety.** Lift the ball higher over the net than usual to allow for any deviation in control, and aim a couple of yards inside the lines. If your opponent comes up to the net, a down-the-line retort is safer, since an errant cross-court attempt could drift the ball into easy hitting range.

5. **Recover quickly.** As soon as you can after the hit, pivot and get back to the court. Don't loop the run to come back in a circular path. Slam on the brakes, then reverse to get back.

THE HALF-VOLLEY

When going up to the net you'll sometimes get caught in a situation where the ball arrives low, at your feet. If you take the ball from flight as it's descending, it will feel like a rock on the strings. You need to compensate with a vice-tight grip and firm forearm to play such a ball. Just be defensive with the shot. Push it back volley-like deep into the court.

Whenever you can, play a safer **half-volley**. That's where you take the ball just after

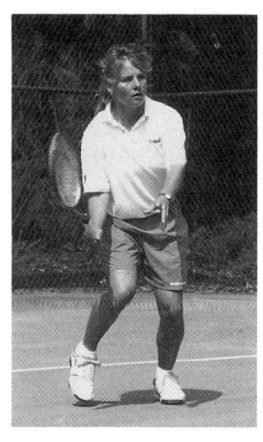

When caught in the middle of the court, the ball often arrives low. Take it with a half-volley; bend your knees . . .

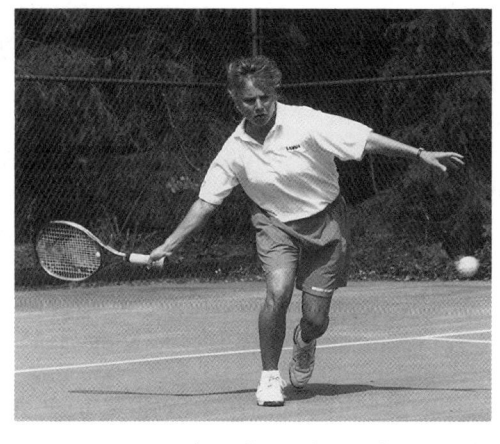

. . . to get extra low; keep the racket parallel with the court, and make contact right after the bounce . . .

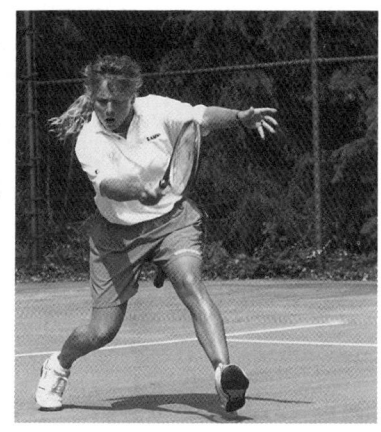

. . . with a forward swing of the racket that makes the act more characteristic of a groundstroke than a volley.

Making Extraordinary Shots Ordinary

its bounce, the way a baseball infielder scoops a ground ball from a short hop. Turn quickly to the side and take only enough backswing to get the racket behind the ball. Meet the ball just an instant after the bounce, with a stable wrist. Tilt the head of the racket back to let the ball carom up and over the net. Bend your knees — lower your seat. Get your head down and try to keep the racket handle parallel to the court. Clear the net with plenty of room. Hit it through a window three feet above the net.

HANDLING A HIGH BACKHAND

The human arm just isn't properly designed to lash into a ball that comes high to the backhand side. Two things will help. First, lift your whole arm up as a unit, keeping it straight. Second, keep the racket at the same angle to your forearm as for an ordinary backhand. Don't try to hit down on the ball. Push the racket out and straight through the ball,

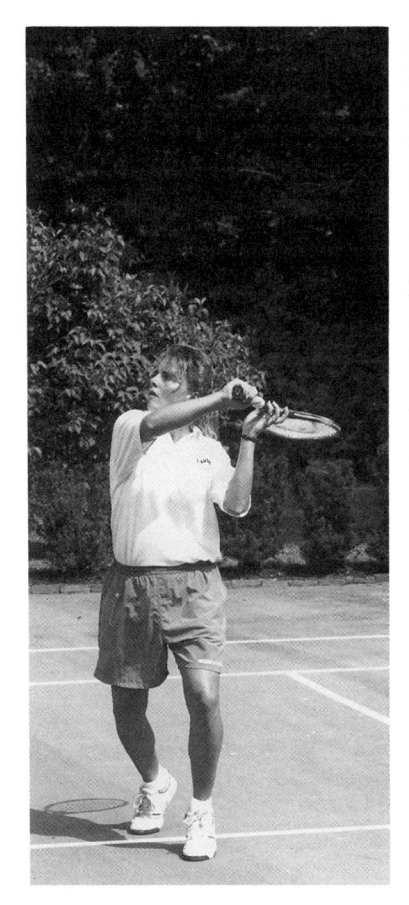

To punch away a high backhand, lift your whole arm, keep it straight . . .

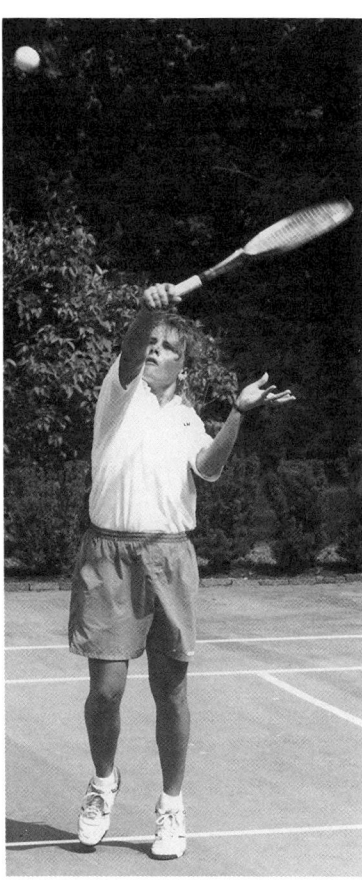

. . . and the wrist laid back, then swat through the ball with the arm held steady.

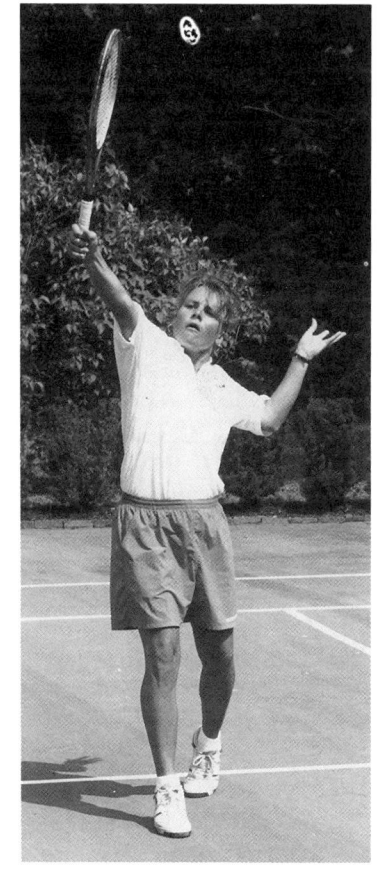

Play it safe. Push the ball back high and deep. Go for control instead of power.

with placement rather than power as the objective.

If you're more confident, rip into a backhand smash. Be sure the ball is high enough to allow your arm to fully extend for the hit. Then get your shoulders turned well around, sideways to the net. Lift your hitting elbow, bend your arm, and cock your wrist to bring the racket back and down, forearm now parallel to the court. Hit by unbending your arm, wrist coming up and over your elbow, and add "whip" to your forearm and wrist for extra pace in the racket head. It's a fairly difficult shot, but if you don't overdo your exuberance when hitting, it can wrest you from an awkward moment and at least keep you alive in the point, if it doesn't win it outright.

RETURNING DEEP LOBS

You're at the net, and an opponent sends a deft lob over your head. You retreat quickly,

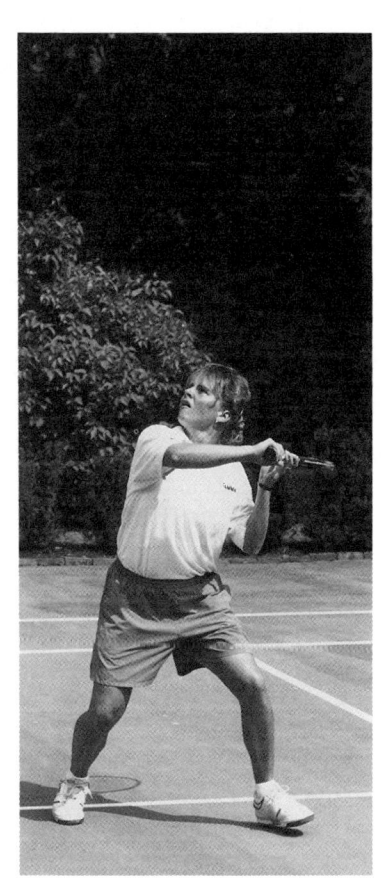

For a backhand smash, get your shoulders turned well round . . .

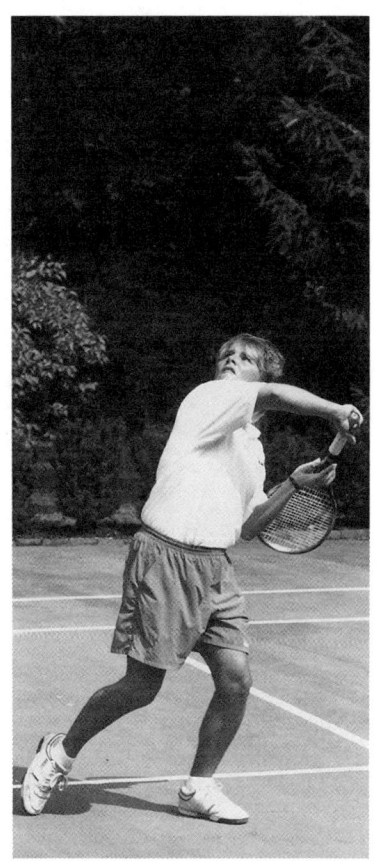

. . . then drop the racket head down and lift your arm up to start a . . .

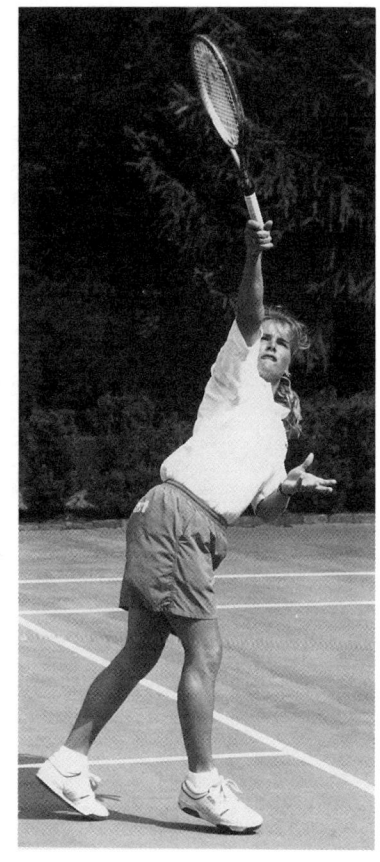

. . . vigorous upward and forward whip of your arm and wrist into the ball.

and catch up to the ball, albeit on a dead run toward the fence.

An offensive return is not possible. So reply with a lob of your own. Return the lob with a lob. Take whatever backswing you can, then lay your racket open and lift your arm upward, coming under the ball to spank it back high. Give your arm a loose-limbed fling, and add some wrist snap to help get the racket moving.

There'll be a tendency to hit too short on this lob, so give the ball plenty of lift and

Suppose you (X) are pushed away from the net by a well-hit offensive lob. Your opponent (O) may follow the shot by taking over the net as you retreat. The safest return is to hit a lob of your own, giving the ball plenty of height and aiming to land it in the middle of your opponent's court.

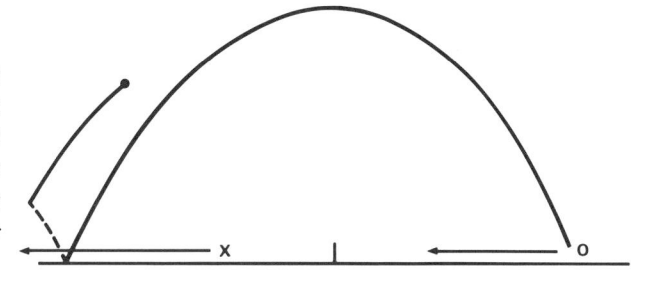

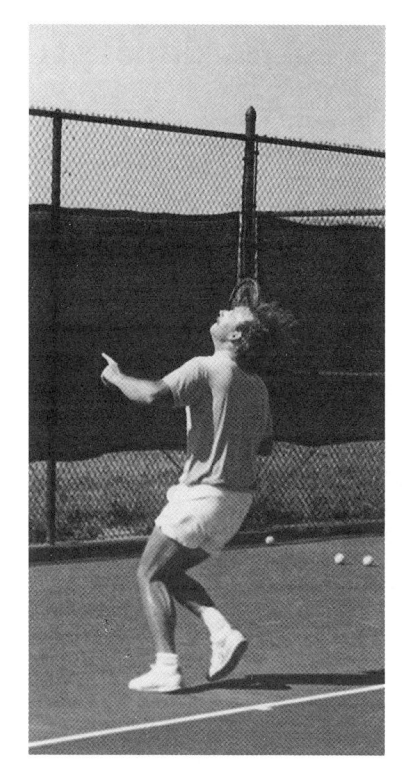

On a full-out retreat to chase down a lob that has bounced and is heading toward the fence . . .

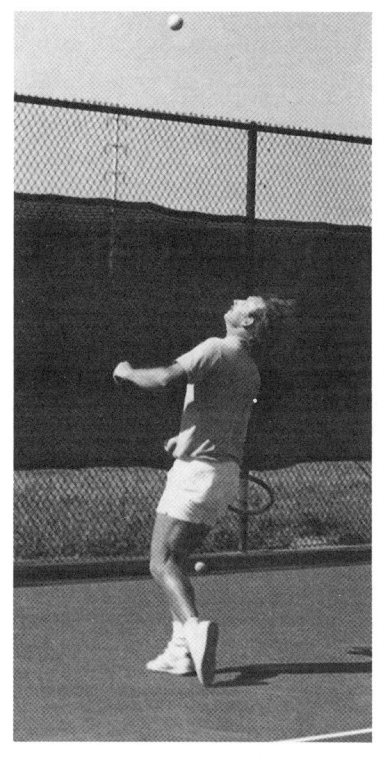

. . . lay the strings toward the sky, take the racket down low, and come up under the ball . . .

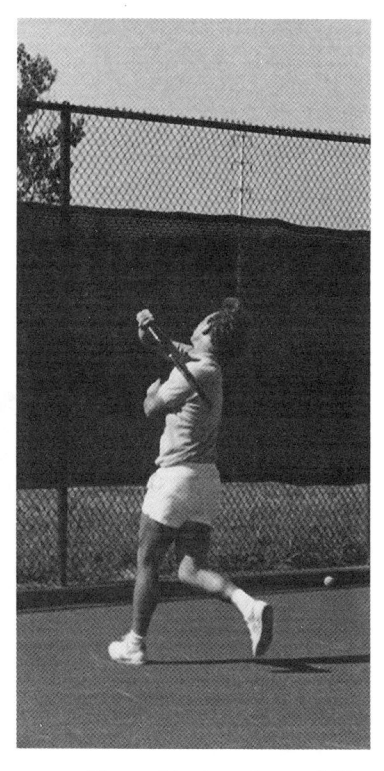

. . . with a whipping skyward fling to get the ball back the best you can. Try for the middle of the court.

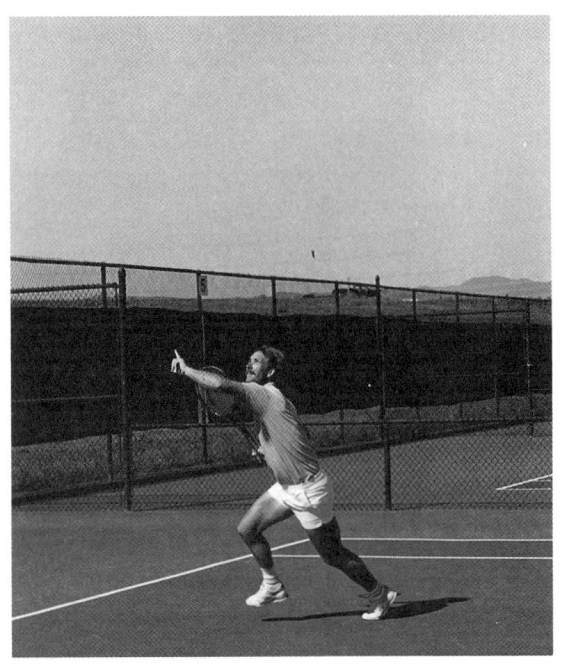

If you can catch up to a lob and get into position for hitting an overhead . . .

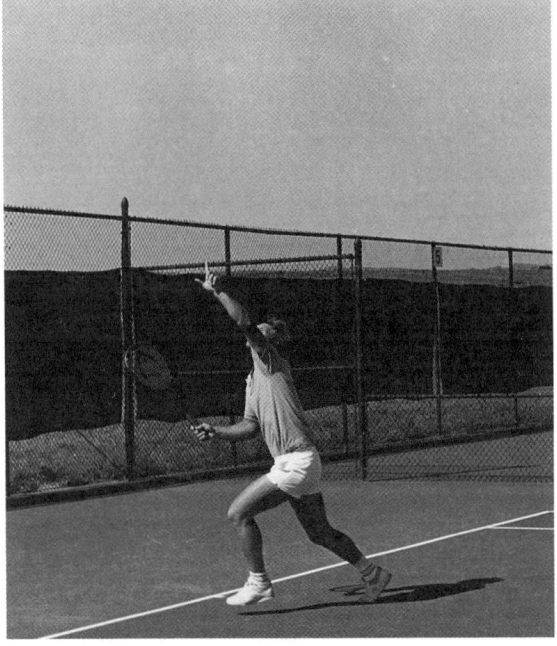

. . . go around behind the ball as much as you can, lift your free arm up to track its path, and . . .

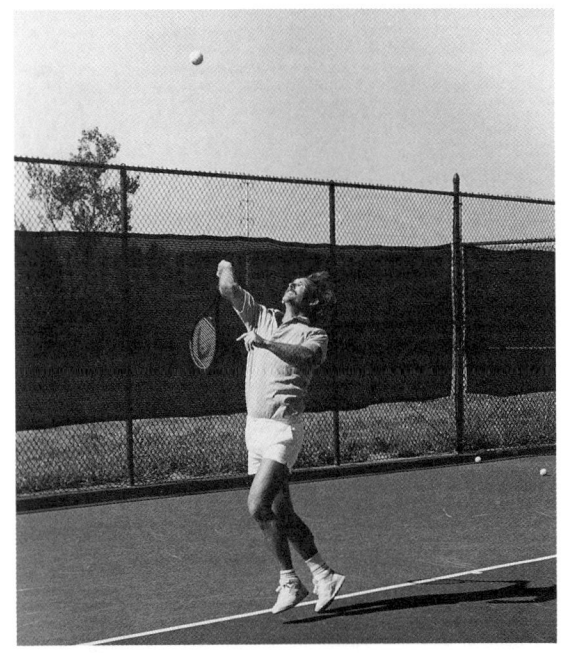

. . . keeping your shoulders turned side-on to the net, get the racket back as for a topspin serve . . .

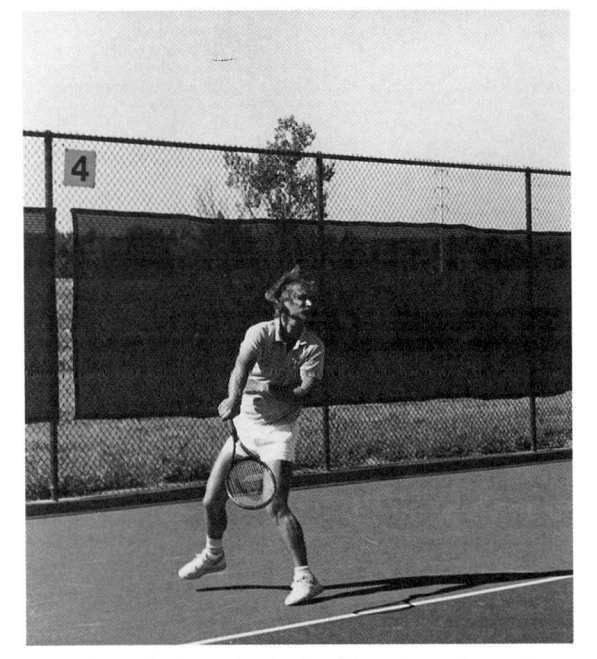

. . . then rip into the ball with a topspin motion, contacting it further back than for a serve.

height. Try to get the ball back to the middle of the court — to the "T" where the service line and center line join. That provides a maximum margin for error in all directions.

Run back parallel to the flight of the ball, but a bit off to the side so that you can swing around your shoulder. Fix your mind on three things: hit the ball back high, hit it to the middle of the court, and don't whack yourself on the head with your follow-through.

In other instances your rival may chase you away from the net with a lob that is high enough to give you time to retreat and get into hitting position. First do what experienced baseball outfielders do when a ball is hit over their head: take a quick sighting of the ball, then turn and run flat-out without bothering to watch its flight. Go well behind the spot where you think the ball will land, then turn and resight the ball again. Make the necessary position adjustments, then hit with a serving-like stroke. Keep your side to the ball. Lift your free arm up toward the ball to guarantee staying sideward and to set your sights on the descending ball. Make the point of contact further back than for a serve, and use a **topspin** motion. If you hit flat on this ball just punch it, but if you give it topspin you can hit with the same freedom you do for a serve, while enjoying the whole court as your target.

USING TOUCH

Moments arise in a match when it's opportune to punch a soft shot, with little pace, away from an opponent. Finesse is the proviso for success. They are the "touch" shots of tennis.

Drop Shot

This return, hit after the ball has bounced, is intended to fall short of a deep opponent. It's generally more workable when played from inside the baseline. But it's a risky shot if it isn't precisely placed, because if it's propelled too far, it becomes a sitter for your opponent.

To play a drop shot, use your normal grip, bring the racket above hitting height and lay the face back, relax your forearm, and push the racket down the back and underneath the ball. Finish low. Ordinarily, the shot should be played against medium paced balls.

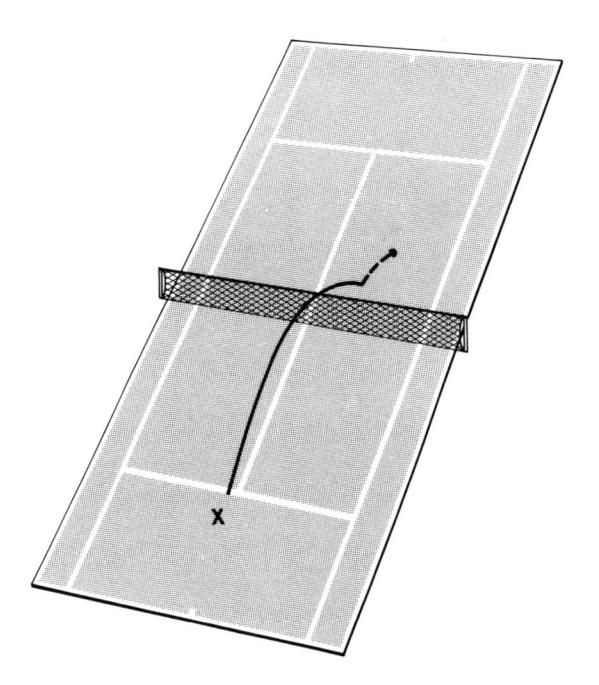

A drop shot is hit just over the net, but only when the opponent is deep behind the baseline. Hit it only when you think you can make it bounce several times before it gets to your opponent's service line. Drive the racket down the back of the ball to give it backspin and further soften the bounce.

Drop Volley

When you're well up in the forecourt and your opponent is deep, you may be able to drop a shallow ball from a volley. The objective is to take the energy out of the ball. There are two ways: either by relaxing your grip almost to the point of letting the racket fall out of your hand and merely allowing the ball to melt into the strings, or by sliding the strings down the back of the ball at contact. Try a combination. Be sure to tilt the racket face back to give some underspin to the ball, but don't let the ball kick too high off the strings where it'll give an opponent time to chase it down. Keep it low over the net.

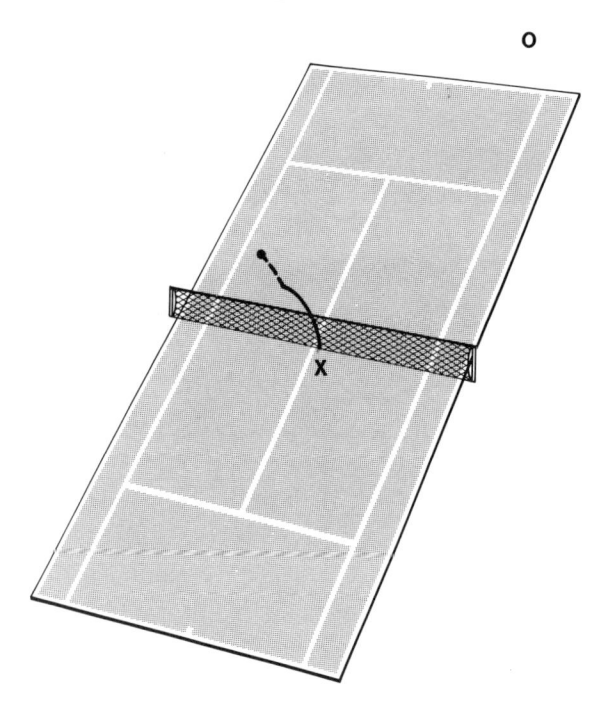

Hit a drop volley only when your opponent is deep, and you're well positioned at the net. Angle the shot away from your rival. Receive the ball like you were catching an egg, but it's your opponent who will be scrambling.

A drop volley can be particularly effective against a fiercely hit drive which you must stretch to reach. Another favorable time is when you've pushed your opponent wide off the court and the return is coming cross-court, giving you lots of vacant area for a target.

Use a drop volley (or a drop shot) only when you're a point or two in the lead, not as a desperation measure. Never chance the shot when you could lose the game if it's unsuccessful. But played at the right time, drop shots can have a demoralizing effect on a tiring opponent.

THE "ANYTHING-GOES" SHOT

The better you get at tennis, and the more aggressively you play, the more you'll find yourself in emergency situations. In many instances, there is no style, only the objective of keeping the ball alive. When you're pressed into awkward shots, use lots of wrist, plenty of fling in the arm, or slap at the ball — just accept your defensive position and do anything to get the ball back. Stay in the point by giving the ball extra height to provide yourself with recovery time. Send it to the middle of the court and, if you can, deep.

BE CREATIVE

To prepare your ready responses for emergencies, during practice try to develop versatility for **all** your strokes. Be creative; experiment with different spins and trajectories, and variations of pace. Learn to hit a wide assortment of shots with the same stroke. For example, make your forehand a reliable weapon for hitting a regular flat drive, or a topspin looper, or with heavy backspin, maybe some slice, and so on. Develop usable modifications for every swing. The more options you have with your strokes, the easier it will be to come up with an answer to distressing circumstances in a match. In the bargain, your practice sessions will be more fun, and during matches you'll hear more grunts of frustration from your opponents when you pull yourself out of desperate situations.

Chapter Eight

Taking Charge of Singles Matches

Sometimes there are night and day differences between the performance in practice and in a game. In the unchallenged free hitting of a practice session, the body may work in smart coordination. But start keeping score, and the muscles might take a vacation.

Often, a lack of competitive confidence comes from a feeling of uncertainty about what to do during a match. And yet, most situations in a game have logical tactical answers. The strategy is remarkably uncomplicated. It all originates from the direct objective of trying to hit the ball so that it cannot be returned or, if returned, is hit so defensively that the point can be won with the next shot. From this all other tactics follow — where to be, where to go, when to go, where to hit the ball, what kind of shot to hit, and so on.

You'll be more relaxed if your approach every match with an attitude of keeping to a simplified plan of strategy. Now is not the time to think of stroke mechanics. Instead, focus on effective strategy, and you'll ease your nervousness.

THE FIRST LAW: KEEP THE BALL IN PLAY

The worst mistake anyone can make is to hit the ball into the net. It's a dead loss, never giving an opponent a chance to make a mistake. Usually it occurs from trying to hit the ball too hard, thus having to skim the net to keep the ball in the court. If this happens, ease up on your stroke to loft the ball more and clear the net with more margin for error.

A related mistake is to hit the ball too wide. This is generally indicative of trying to rifle an angled shot too near the sideline. Always aim several feet inside the lines, where there's allowance for some inaccuracy.

Hit the ball over the net, land it in-bounds, and do this one more time than your opponent. It is the first law of strategy.

THE SECOND LAW: KEEP THE BALL DEEP

An associated tactic is to place the ball deep. This will compel an opponent into staying back, hitting incessantly from behind the baseline with little chance to come up to the net and with reduced opportunities for hitting angled, cross-court returns. You'll also provide yourself with more time for moving into ideal hitting position on each ball, thus allowing preparation for a rhythmical, forward-flowing swing.

During practice, monitor your rally to try to consistently land the ball behind the opposing service line, and preferably within a yard or two of the baseline. Become sensitive to how hard you can hit the ball and still keep it in-bounds.

KNOW WHEN TO USE ANGLES

When your opponent offers a shallow ball, one that you can play from inside the baseline, then be ready to take advantage of cross-court angles. The most favorable opportunity is when you get a return that is both shallow and off to one side. Then your rival's court has added width, for you can either fling a cross-court winner in front of your opponent, or plunk the ball into the near corner behind your surprised adversary. Of the two choices, the cross-court shot is generally safer.

From behind your own baseline, you are usually left with only the choice of hitting the ball deep. But when you get an inviting short ball:

1. the further inside the court you can move to retrieve the ball, the greater the potential for angling a shot toward either sideline. But,
2. the more you are pulled off to one **side** of your own court, the more favorable the situation becomes for a **cross-court** return.

Even if you are behind your own baseline — but still off to one side — a cross-court shot is generally a more logical choice than a down-the-line placement because:

1. the distance to the opposite diagonal corner is greater than the distance to the near corner, thus providing more room for placement;
2. the ball will cross the net near the middle, where the net is six inches lower than at the sides;
3. the ball will be moving away from your opponent, whereas a down-the-line shot will swing the ball back toward your rival, and;

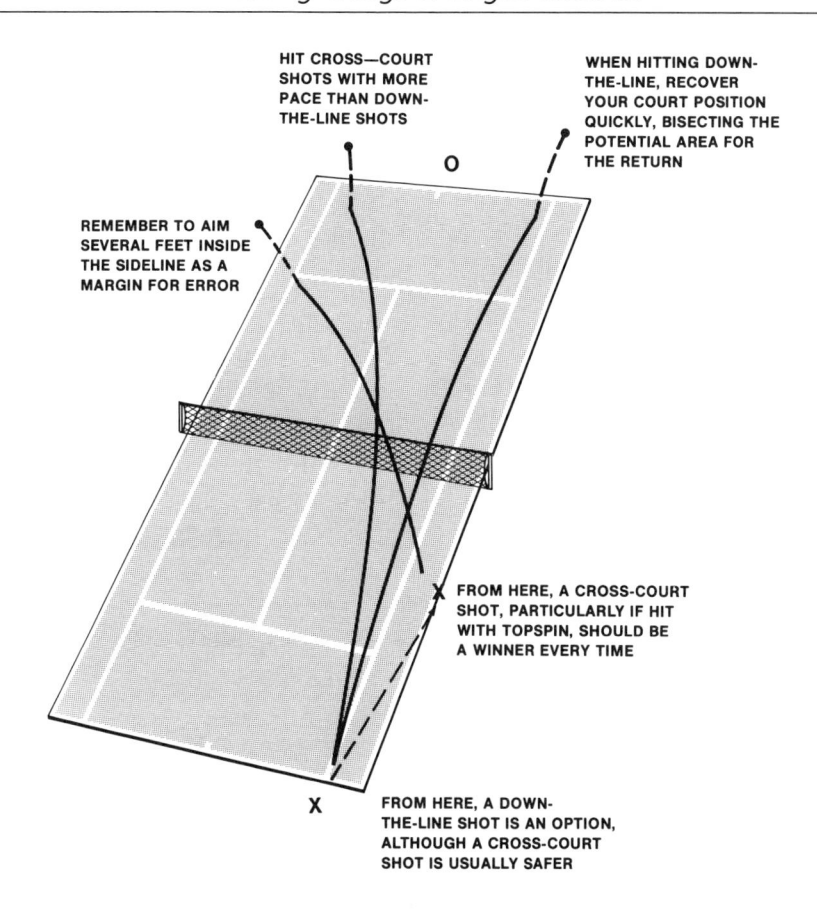

Using angles from a sideline position.

4. you are in better position following the shot to cover the potential area of your opponent's return.

HOW TO BEAT A STRONG GROUNDSTROKE PLAYER

In a match against a player who can effectively produce well-placed groundstrokes, consider keeping the deep in the **middle** of the court. Tradition has it that you should run a groundstroke player from side to side, presumably to force them into off-balance shots. But sometimes, the last thing you want to do is to provide this player with opportunities for hitting angled shots that keep you scampering for returns.

It is especially vital to keep the ball deep and in the middle of the court if your adversary can hit topspin. Against such a player, an unforgiving mistake is to hit a ball shallow and to the side, where it is an open invitation for a cross-court winner.

IF YOUR OPPONENT IS A SLUGGER

Playing a big hitter is a challenge to your reflexes. They can control the fate of every point, either by winning them outright or by losing them on errors. And therein lies their destiny. Sluggers are often impatient. If they haven't won a point after a few exchanges, they become more aggressive and hit a shot with a higher probability of failure. Few power hitters can follow one great shot with a consecutive series of others. So observe the first law of tennis: keep the ball in play.

Additionally, a big hitter likes to have the ball come to them with good pace. It's more difficult to generate power off a ball that does not itself have much impulse. So offer this player a "nothing" ball. Take some strength out of your returns to float the ball back with good net clearance, and land it deep. Use backspin to slow the ball both in flight and after its bounce. This compels the slugger into a slower timed swing, and their out-of-rhythm mechanics will force more mistakes.

Control the sequence of the exchange by hitting hard, then slow, then deep, then short. Get the ball back at any cost. Loop it,

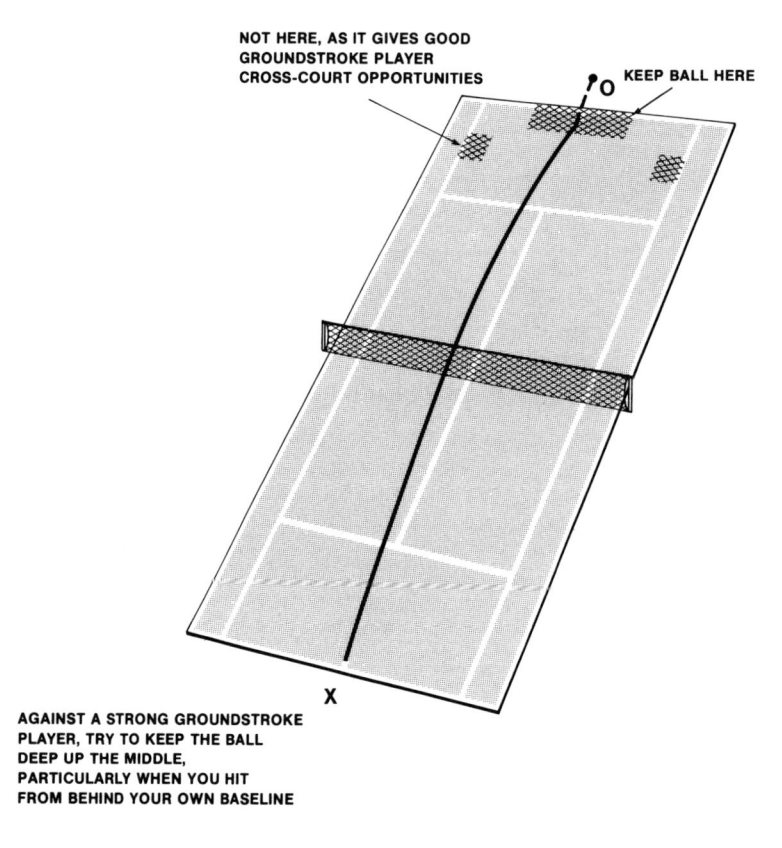

NOT HERE, AS IT GIVES GOOD GROUNDSTROKE PLAYER CROSS-COURT OPPORTUNITIES

KEEP BALL HERE

AGAINST A STRONG GROUNDSTROKE PLAYER, TRY TO KEEP THE BALL DEEP UP THE MIDDLE, PARTICULARLY WHEN YOU HIT FROM BEHIND YOUR OWN BASELINE

Playing against a strong groundstroke opponent.

lob it, loft it. The overall objective is depth, where the slugger's frustration will be your satisfaction.

There are times, however, when a big hitter should be brought up to the net. Smashball players often prefer to crush the ball from their own baseline, and may feel uncomfortable at the net, where touch and finesse are necessary.

Find out by dropping some trial shots just over the net. Backspin these shots, for if they are mistakenly hit too deep, the halting action of the bounce will still make it more difficult for the power player to get their full weight into the swing.

Get as many first serves in as you can because a strong hitter will be looking to pulverize the second. Go for an occasional big second serve when you have the lead. Spin a high percentage of the serves wide to pull the power player off the court and stretch them out laterally where they cannot set up to unwind their swing. The same is true for ground strokes. When you hit your own shot with good pace, push your opponent off the court so they cannot get planted and comfortable to unleash a buggy-whip swing. Wrong-foot them often by hitting the ball to the area they just came from. If they are especially strong on the forehand side, keep the ball away from that side on crucial points (0-30; 15-40, etc.).

IF YOUR OPPONENT IS A HUMAN BACKBOARD

If you're up against a player who scrambles to return every ball — although often with little pace — the ploy of keeping the ball alive will have less effect. Consistent baseline players have confidence in their own ability to keep the ball in play and will not likely become impatient during a prolonged exchange. But they are also less apt to try for put-away shots, so moving these players from side to side will not invite the cross-court winners that it does from big hitters.

Add extra pace to your shots. A steady baseline player often hits defensively, so your extra pace will increase the chances of getting a shallow return that allows you to step into the court and take advantage of the angles. You'll also have more opportunity to approach the net, as the slower ball from the defensive player will give you more time to make the trip. Be wary that your backboard-like opponent may have good command of the lob. But if you do the preliminary work of sending the approach shot deep, your rival's potential for an effective offensive lob is reduced, and it's unlikely you'll get passed by a strong drive hit out of your reach.

USE THE FORECOURT OFTEN

One mark of a confident, aggressive player is an instinct for coming up to the net at every opportunity. Against some opponents, when you show an intent to make frequent use of the forecourt, you inflict a plaguing mental diversion that constantly interferes with their concentration. They'll keep an apprehensive eye on you and will hit more cautiously to try to keep you in the backcourt. And when you do come to the net, your very presence alone may be enough to press a jittery opponent into committing unforced errors.

If you hit an approach shot from near the sideline, it's marginally safer to hit cross-court, but this also opens up an inviting area of your own court for your opponent. Consequently, the better choice may be to hit down-the-line. This will make it easier to cover the widest possible angles that your opponent will have for the return. If you prefer a cross-court approach shot, use it more often when you can leave the open court on your stronger side.

Go to the net as often as you can, even if you're still uncertain about the logic. Each trip will add to your confidence. Generate an attitude of **always** looking for a chance to move forward. Productive groundstroke play is essentially a matter of keeping the ball alive until your adversary offers a shallow return. Then, take the invitation and step up to the net.

HIT THE BALL WHERE YOUR OPPONENT ISN'T

Once at the net, the intent is to win the point as soon as possible. Hit the ball someplace — anyplace — where it's not likely to be returned.

There's an old baseball adage about how to be a successful batter: "Hit the ball where the fielders aren't." The principle is the same for net play in tennis. Fling the ball someplace where you opponent cannot reach it.

It's the same for the overhead, but for this shot don't be too precise with the placement. Let the force of the shot command much of the influence.

AGAINST A NET RUSHER

Nobody's perfect. Occasionally you drop a ball too shallow, and your assailant takes the net. Now let your rival's approach shot tell you what to do.

If the ball comes deep, forcing you to hit from behind the baseline, the logical retort is to lift a lob over your opponent's backhand shoulder. Make it an offensive lob if you can, since some players will rush the net flat out and you can therefore float the ball just over their reach. Otherwise, if their approach shot comes up short, the further in you can move to play the ball, the more the percentage turns in favor of a passing shot. If you are pressed toward the sideline, hit the ball down-the-line so it will get to the net-rusher more quickly. If you're in the middle of the court, hit the passing shot to either side, aiming to land it near the intersection of the service line and the sideline. Such placement may resolve the point right away, or at least force the on-rushing player to lunge for the ball and drop the racket down to reply with a more defensive shot.

HIT SHOTS IN SEQUENCE

If tennis is like chess, to which it is often likened, then one of the similarities is the sequential pattern of play. Both require patience and a plot for openings. One move leads to another in a logical, planned order.

The first ploy in chess-like tennis is to find the right moment to maneuver your opponent to one side of the court. This sets up a chance to fling the ball behind your

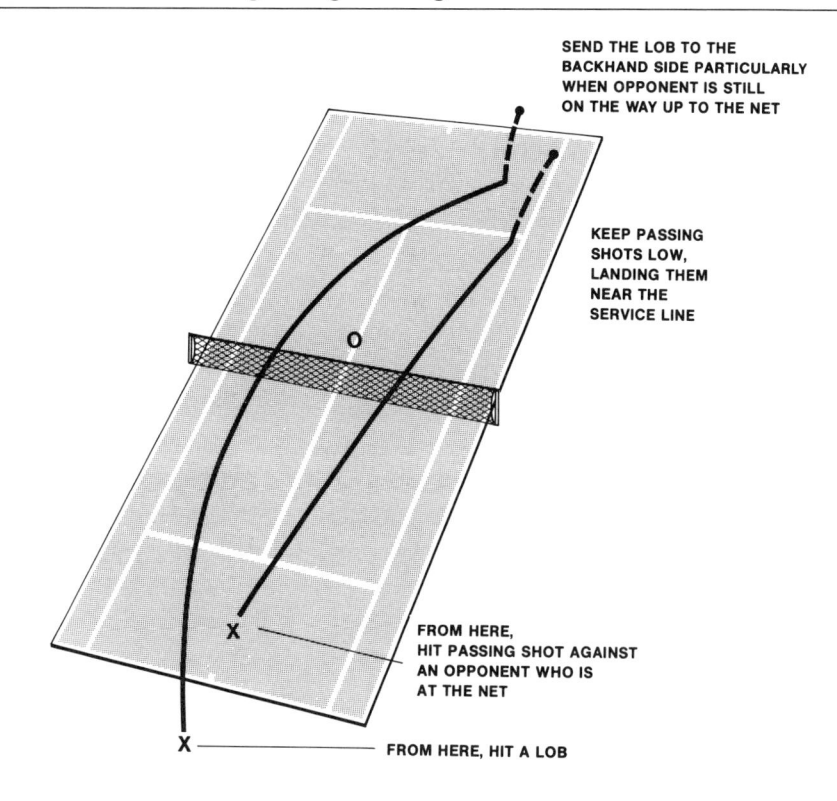

Playing (as "x") against an opponent ("o") who is at the net.

rival, into the area of the court they just vacated, and with a well-paced shot you can win the point directly, or at least force a feeble return that lets you pounce on the next ball for a put-away.

A frequently suggested sequence of shots is the "up-and-back" philosophy: drive your opponent deep behind the baseline, then lay a drop shot just over the net to catch your rival stranded too far back to retrieve the shallow ball. The weak link in this cycle is the drop shot, for unless it's deftly hit, it could become a sitter for an angled, point winning return. Another variation, usually safer, is to start the sequence by hitting deep into a corner (especially when you can do this with a cross-court shot), then follow with a short placement along the opposite sideline. This makes a longer run for your opponent, and even if the ball is chased down it will probably be from a sprint that produces only a weak return and leaves a wide open court for your next shot. If you initiate this sequence of shots by first hitting into your opponent's forehand corner you should have your mind focused on a short follow-up shot. But if you hit first into the backhand corner you can expect a subdued reply which could be a candidate for a rousing crack at an aggressive winner. In fact, any

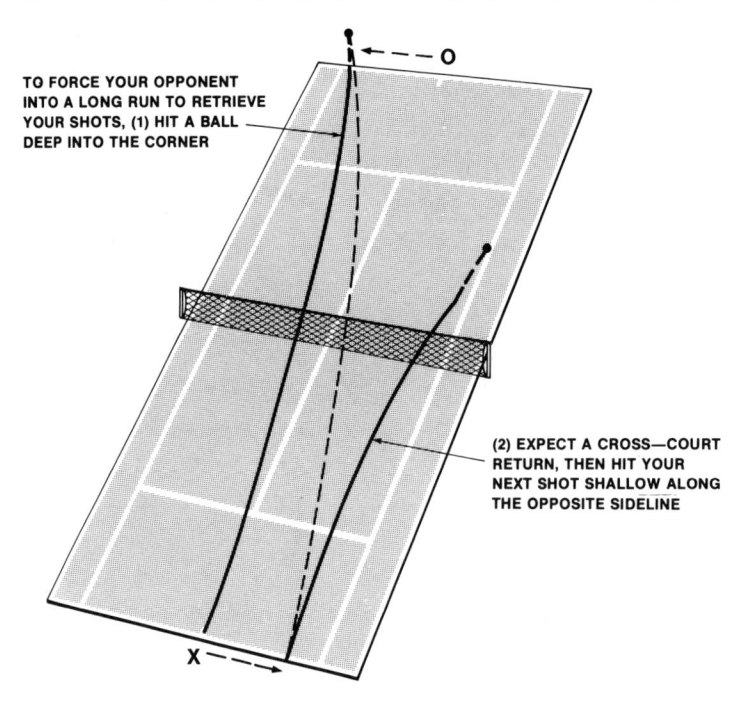

Hitting a deep-corner and shallow-side sequence of shots.

ball which is hit deep into your opponent's back hand corner should heighten your readiness to move in and catch the return early for an angled put-away.

MAKE THINGS HAPPEN

The overall objective of playing a series of chess-like shots is to create some activity. It is to cause events rather than waiting for things to happen. Thus, by variable ball placement you can take the offensive, compelling an opposing player into hitting off-balance returns and increasing the chances of extracting an error.

You can do much the same by varying the pace and spin of the ball, or by adding extra velocity to your shots to induce defensive returns. Always, the intent is to do something that will make an opponent respond to **your** actions rather you to theirs. It will create openings and allow you to be more opportunistic. And you'll have more influence over the outcome of points.

Don't be overzealous, however. If you get pressured into a defensive predicament, accept your fate and respond with a defensive return. But even when you're hitting defensively, you can still be working for the advantage. Sometimes it's enough just to stay in a point by scrambling to get the ball back any way you can. Or if the momentum of an exchange of shots has put you on your heels, try lifting the next ball higher over the net than usual, even as a semi-lob. At some instant the momentum will change, even from a purely defensive return, and you'll regain the offensive again.

FOR THE LEFT-HANDERS

Are you left-handed? If so the rotation of the earth combined with the Coriolis Effect combined with your spin gives you a force-vector advantage. Seriously. So you should hit lots of slice on your serves and topspin on your ground strokes. The effect is to send right-handers into gyrational disarray.

For the rest of us mortals who are right-handed we already know that the ball comes off a lefty's racket with wrong-way rotation. So we could vow to play a left-hander only in the southern hemisphere, where the earth-effect is the opposite, or we must change the direction of our shots to send the ball incessantly to the backhand side of the left-hander to stop their traffic of topspin forehands that kick into our body. This gives the right-handed player lots of chances to hit cross-court forehands, which should be a more natural direction to send the ball anyhow. And keep almost all the backhand returns down-the-line.

When your left-handed opponent hits topspin off the forehand, step around your backhand more often to hit more of your own forehands. That's to counteract the effect of the oncoming ball which, after its bounce, will jump into the body of a player preparing for a backhand.

The most distraught time is when a left-hander hits heavy spin on the serves. On the forehand side it moves into the right-hander's body. On the backhand side it swerves further and further away. To reduce this effect, stand in an extra step or two when receiving to take the ball earlier. The later you take it, the more effective the spin.

PLAY WITHIN YOUR ABILITY

It is sometimes tempting, when the opportunity arises, to try to pull off a dazzling point winner with an unusual miracle shot. But probably you've never practiced such shots. Therefore, it's better to hit shots you know you own. Keep your technique within your ability. This is especially vital in two circumstances: when you have an easy put-away, and when you are playing critical points. The first instance draws on emotion rather than skill. When your opponent offers a sitter, it's tempting to hit with more-than-necessary force, as if to make some kind of declaration of dominance. But missing an easy shot leaves you with an agonizing feeling of disbelief, while the opponent can be rejuvenated by the reprieve. So do only what is necessary to win these easy points.

Relatedly, do not try unusual shots on big points. A drop shot is an example — it needs fine touch, a small area of effective placement, and the right opportunity. If it's poorly hit, it's either netted or becomes an easy setup for the opponent. Therefore, with such risk factors, do not try such surprise shots when you are playing a crucial point (as, for example, when you could lose the game off that point). Save them for the middle of a game, when you still have time to recover if they fail.

GET THE FIRST SERVE IN

All too often players assume they should crush their first serve and, if not successful, push the second. Instead, it would be well to slow down the first serve and increase the pace of the second.

First serves should be made good on at least half the attempts, mainly to keep the opponent from hitting from behind the baseline. In addition, a first serve that can be consistently hit in-bounds is a great psychological boost that adds spirit and confidence to your entire game. Moreover, the most opportune time for coming to the net will be behind first rather than second serves.

Analyze your second serve not so much by whether it's hit in-bounds, but rather by how often it wins points. For instance, if you are successful on nearly all your second serves but find that you are losing more than half the points, it could be that your second attempts are too slow, allowing opponents to step up and hit winners. Therefore, you need to risk a lower percentage of successful placement by hitting the second serves harder, thus forcing your opponents to be more defensive, and in the process boosting your point-winning percentages off these serves.

In reality, you never need to hit any serve harder than necessary to win points. If you find that your opponent cannot handle even your second serves, then slow down your first serves to make them good more often, thereby further reducing any risk of double faults.

WHERE TO HIT THE SERVE

There are basically three areas for placement of the serve: (1) the far corners, (2) the near corners, and (3) directly at the receiver.

1. Serves hit to the **far corner** in either court will pull the receiver wide and open up a roomy area for a volley of the return. When hit to the far corner of the ad court, the serve not only drags the receiver wide, it also attacks the weaker side (of a right-handed player) and thus presents the best opportunity to follow the serve into the forecourt in anticipation of a soft return.
2. Serves hit **down-the-middle** have the benefit of reducing the receiver's potential to hit cross-court returns. And, since these placements bring the receiver to the middle of the court, a charge to the net following the serve will have less vulnerability to an angled return.
3. When the serve is hit **directly at the receiver**, it may force that player to waste a fatal microsecond deciding whether to take the ball with a forehand or a backhand. Besides, a ball coming directly at someone is more difficult to judge for flight characteristics than one that can be seen at an angle. When using topspin, direct the ball just off-center toward the receiver's backhand. The curving arc of the ball will bring it into a difficult spot: tight on the forehand side, thus forcing an awkward response and virtually assuring a weak return (and favoring a net charge).

Second serves should be hit to the weaker side of the receiver more often than first serves. And try to hit all serves **deep**. Except when hitting exaggerated topspin to intentionally land the ball shallow along the sideline (see diagram), a short ball will otherwise allow the receiver to wrest the attacking initiative away from you. Especially on second serves, the reliability of depth must come from its controlling spin and downward flight, rather than a cautious shallow placement.

Experiment with standing at different distances from the center mark. Kick serves hit to the corners or along the sideline will swerve wider if you stand off-center. When standing out wide to serve into the ad court, a serve to the corner will almost assuredly come back to your forehand side.

Take the net behind the serve often, especially when you hit extra spin, for the higher, dipping path of the ball will give you more time to advance. Charge directly along the flight of your serve where you'll be in the middle of the possible angles for its return.

If your opponent gets a good quality return of your serve it will come back fast and low. Make sure you punch through the ball on your first volley to hit it deep into a corner. Then finish your charge to the net, always directly behind the path of your shot. If the ball comes back yet another time, try

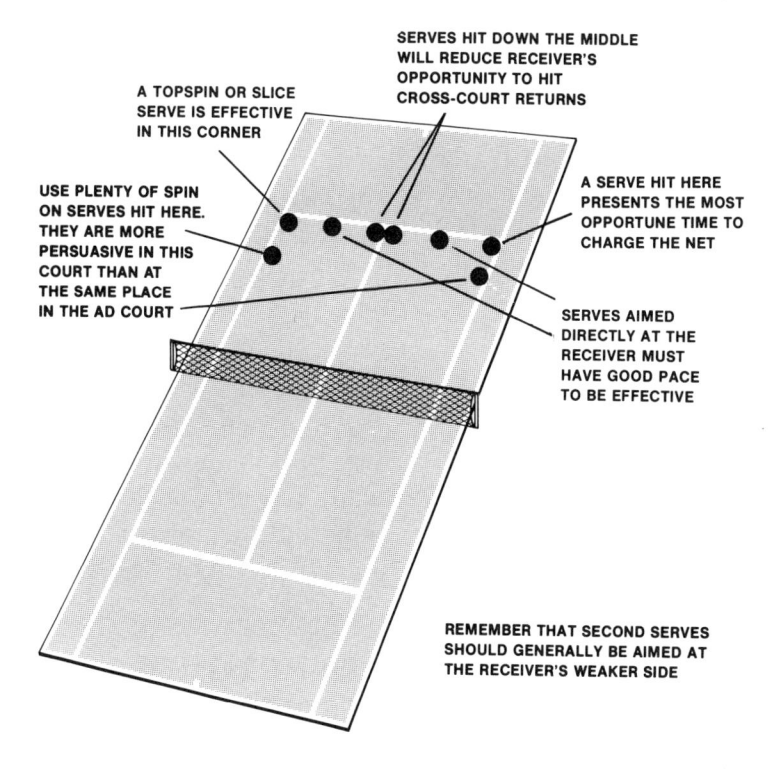

Placement choices for the serve.

to end the rally with the next shot by angling it out of reach.

ATTACK THE SECOND SERVE

When receiving the serve, first clear your mind of any thoughts about being in a defensive position. Instead, think of **attacking**. Breaking your opponent's serve gives you a colossal advantage of the psyche. It's incredibly demoralizing for an opposing player when you take control of the games they serve.

Best time to attack is on the second serve. Most players do not hit forceful second serves, so stand in front of the baseline, take the ball on the rise, and drive it down-the-line. If it's well hit, charge the net behind your return. On short, weak serves, run around your backhand to crush an offensive return from your stronger side. The second serve may be the shortest ball you'll see during a match. Take advantage of it by drilling the ball back and instantaneously shifting the momentum of the point to your side of the net.

BEAT THE ELEMENTS

Don't let it rain on your game. If you're playing in a drizzle or mist or in high humidity, the ball gets heavy and must be hit harder. By contrast, in hot, dry weather the ball travels faster and bounces higher, so topspin your shots more often to bring them down and kick them high. Hit fewer shots with underspin than you normally would.

If the sun is a problem when serving on one end, toss the ball further back over your head and adjust by hitting more spin. Lob more often when the sun is at your back to use its distracting glare for your opponent.

If there is a wind at your back, arc your serves and groundstrokes with extra topspin. When serving into the wind toss the ball lower to flatten the serve for more power and less spin, and stay back in anticipation of a deep return. On groundstrokes, with the wind at your back, take a shorter backswing but follow-through normally. Go to the net often. When hitting into the wind, take the topspin off your groundstrokes to hit flat, penetrating shots. Lob deep when your opponent comes in behind their own wind-aided approach shots. If there is a crosswind, the confusing current could make the ball swerve at the last instant, so use stutter steps as you approach the ball for final adjustments in hitting position. Hit crosscourt into the wind, but keep away from angled shots when the wind might pick up the ball and float it wide.

When playing under the lights, shorten your backswing on groundstrokes and especially on service returns because the lower visibility will make the ball seem to come at you more quickly. Lob more often to make the ball disappear momentarily into the lights. Come to the net less often because it's more difficult to track a high speed return and hit an effective volley.

ADAPT TO THE COURT SURFACE

The soft, granular surface of "slow" courts will grab the ball on the bounce, slowing it down and making it rebound higher. Consequently, the biggest adjustment is to anticipate longer rallies. Therefore:

1. Play more patiently, keeping the ball alive, trying less frequently for put-aways, and being more selective about going to the net.
2. Spin is more effective on slow surfaces. Use topspin often, particularly on serves. But wide serves will not slide off the side of the court as much as on a fast court, so slice serves will be less influential.
3. Slow down the first serves to get them in more often, since aces are less likely and power is less compelling. Also, it gives the receiver less chances to attack the court-slowed second serve.
4. Keep groundstrokes deep, with topspin, to discourage opponents from coming to the net.
5. Since footing is less sure, make your opponents change directions often. Use angled shots and touch shots, and hit the ball behind your rival more often. Use more changes in pace to keep opponents from maintaining the rhythm that is more easily acquired on slow courts.

On hard-surface courts, the play is faster because of the tendency of the ball to skid and stay low after the bounce. Accordingly, it's more important to make things happen rather than trying to wear an opponent down.

1. Footing is more sure, so come around the ball to get into ideal hitting position and put more weight into each shot. Be aggressive with the groundstrokes. Go for the open court more often.
2. Because the ball does not slow down as much from the bounce, prepare your racket earlier and shorten the backswing, especially when returning serves.
3. Attack the net more often to put added pressure on your opponent. Go in behind your serve and on your opponent's second serve.
4. Hit strong serves. Use a flat serve more often, and slice the ball to the far corner of the deuce court where it will pull an opponent especially wide.
5. Use backspin more frequently on driving groundstrokes, since it will make the ball skid and will pave your way up to the net.

PLAY PERCENTAGE TENNIS

In the final analysis, logical strategy is a matter of percentages. Shot selection should be based on the probability of success at any given moment, or at least on keeping you in the point. It means doing what makes sense, and the guiding principles are:

- What do you do best?
- What does your opponent do worst?

It its simplest form, strategy is a process of linking the two together. Does your opponent have a weak backhand? Play to it often. Do **you** have a weak backhand? Run around it often. If you are confident with flat serves, hit flat serves. Use your strengths. Exploit your opponents' vulnerabilities. That way you'll **win** instead of having avoided losing.

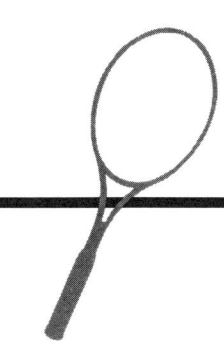

Chapter Nine

Strategic Strength for Doubles

Good doubles play merely requires lightening-fast reflexes, winged feet, quick hands, uncanny finesse, unfailing accuracy, extrasensory anticipation, infinite fortitude, and unshakable nerves. In general, it's a game of position, patience, and placement.

1. **Position:** The over-riding objective of doubles is to gain control of the net, from where most of the points are won.
2. **Patience:** The doubles court is only nine feet wider than the singles court, but with twice as many players protecting it, the points are not so likely to end after only one or two shots.
3. **Placement:** There's a premium on accuracy. Singles is a game of speed; doubles is a game of precision.

Played poorly, doubles can be a drag. But played well it's a fiery game of dexterity and cooperation between partners.

GET A GOOD START

At the start of each set, the stronger server of the two partners should serve first, without exception. This does not necessarily mean the hardest server, but rather the player whose accuracy and pace best suits the tactics of doubles play.

When receiving, the steadier and/or stronger player normally takes the ad court, since that's where the most crucial points are played. Additionally, the ad-court player usually hits more shots in a match because of having the right-of-way to return balls arriving up the middle (to the forehand of that player). If one player is left-handed and the other right-handed, the lefty should usually take the ad court so that both players can return wide angled shots with forehands.

SERVING STRATEGY

If your first serve is not too reliable, decrease its strength to get it in more often, mainly to keep the receiver from having too many chances to take the second ball and tattoo it onto the forehead of your net-playing partner. Deliver the first serves with less speed and more spin than normal. If you have command of topspin, use it almost exclusively. Hit to the backhand of the receiver more often than in singles, because:

1. The return will probably be slower, giving your partner more time to respond with a winning volley.
2. The slower paced return allows more time for the server to approach the net.
3. The return itself is far less likely to be a sinking low drive hit at the feet of a net-charging server.

Serve from a position away from the center mark so you're ready to cover your half of the court. Then approach the net by going straight forward instead of following on-line directly behind the path of the served ball as in singles.

THE SERVER'S PARTNER

The partner of the server should stand midway between the center line and the doubles sideline. Forget any neurotic compulsion to protect the alley. Few receivers will be talented enough to send the ball back along the doubles sideline. Get out into the court where the return is more likely to be hit. You'll be a more menacing figure there, and even if you do tempt a receiver to hit behind you, that player will have been coerced into aiming for a narrow target.

Have the attitude of an aggressive soccer goalie. Go after the ball at every reasonable opportunity. You have first rights to every shot that comes back. Take advantage of your position to punch an angled winner on every low return, or smash every lob you can effectively reach.

POACHING, AND OTHER FAKERY

Poaching is when the net player on the serving team trespasses over into the empty area on the other side of the court in anticipation of intercepting a cross-court return. It's best to wait until the receiver is committed — when they can no longer change their mind about where the ball is going to be hit. Then **go**! Quickly! Take the ball early. Shove it right down at the feet of the receiver's partner (if that player is at the net) or volley it out of reach if both are back at the baseline.

Another effective tactic is to fake a poach. In this case you **want** the receiver to notice

Strategic Strength for Doubles 109

The diagram to the right shows the server's starting position in doubles (which should be closer to the sideline than in singles) and the proper straight-ahead line of approach to the net following the serve. When the serve is hit into the far corner, as illustrated, the net player should take a quick step toward the sideline to protect the alley.

In the photo below, the straight-ahead approach of the server shows that it maintains optimal court coverage, while the receiver in this case has performed the appropriate tactic of hitting the return away from the net player, back toward the server.

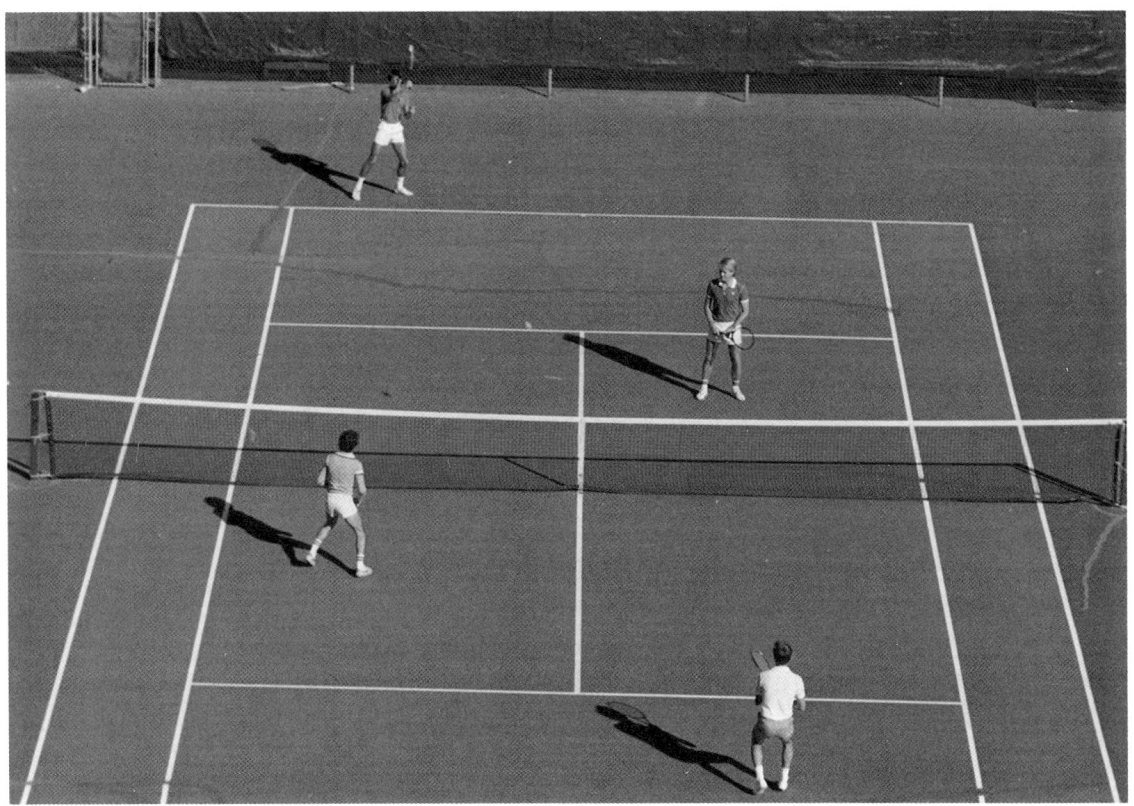

you, so start a simulated poach early, while the serve is still on its way. Use a head and shoulder movement like a basketball player driving toward the goal. Make the receiver see this fake, and it may lure them into taking their eyes off the ball or changing their point of aim in midswing. Hold your ground and expect a weaker return to come right at you for an easy volley.

Remember that your own partner, the server, must know when you will poach. As you cross over, the server is obliged to cover your emptied side of the court. It's a scissors act, net player poaching and server shifting behind the net player's original position. Commonly, before the serve, the net player will show the plan to the server by a hand signal, held behind the back to conceal it from the opponents. A closed fist, for example, could mean the net player will stay, while an open hand would mean there will be a poach.

Poaching is the caper of tennis. It gives the two of you more of a sense of being a team — of having planned moves. And it's also intimidating to opponents. After you do it a few times early in a match, you'll find the receivers being hesitant with their returns. The best time to pull it off is when the serve is hit down the middle in the deuce court, to the receiver's backhand, and therefore the server should keep that as the aim point on a poach. But try it often, on different serves. Then, even when you don't poach, the threat of it will force the receiver to keep a wary eye on you, and the shellshocked partner of the receiver will no longer take up an offensive position at the net during the serve.

RETURNING THE SERVE

There are two objectives for returning the serve in doubles:

1. Get the ball past the net player.
2. Keep the ball low enough so that the server cannot ram it back for a winner.

Generally, this means hitting a cross-court return, either driven right at the shoestrings of a net-charging server, or aimed at the singles sideline if the server stays back. But if

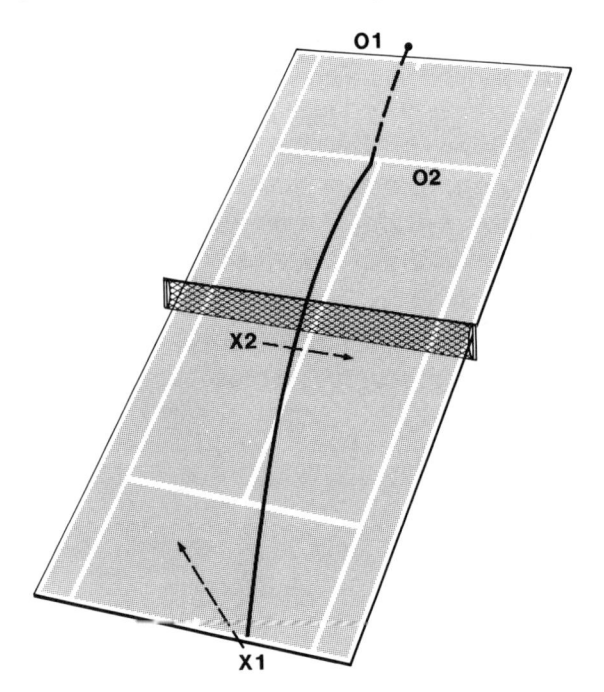

A poach often produces its best results when the serve is hit down-the-middle in the deuce court, where it attacks the receiver's backhand and eliminates any possibility of a sharply angled return. Then, as the net player (X2) poaches and the server (X1) covers the vacated space, both players are positioned for any return.

Strategic Strength for Doubles

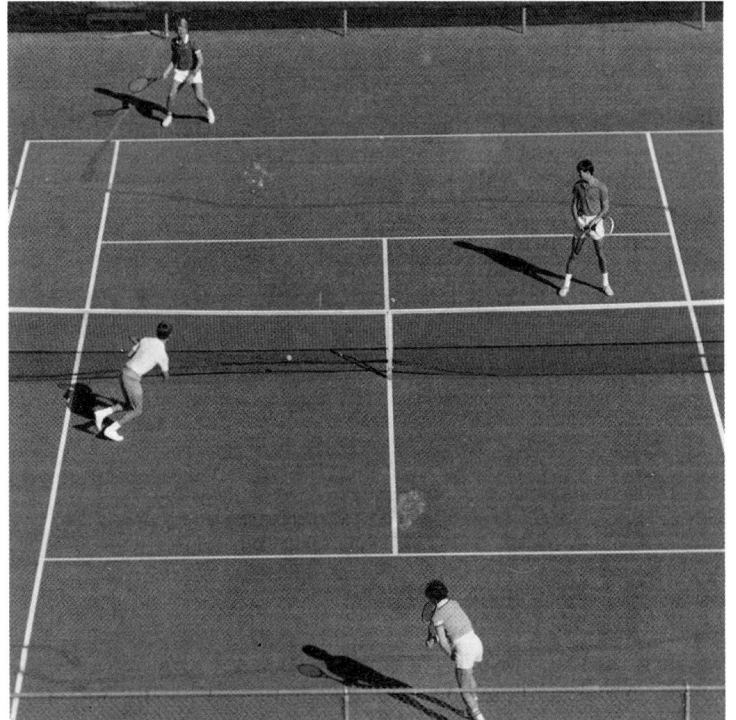

Here's the poach in motion. The server's partner has started to cross the court, while the server moves over to cover the net player's side of the court. The net player must signal the plan to the server prior to the serve so the scissors act can be coordinated.

In general, it's best to return the serve, whenever possible, toward the intersection of the singles sideline and the service line, where it will either be low and away from an onrushing server, or it might be an outright winner by passing out-of-reach of a server who does not charge the net.

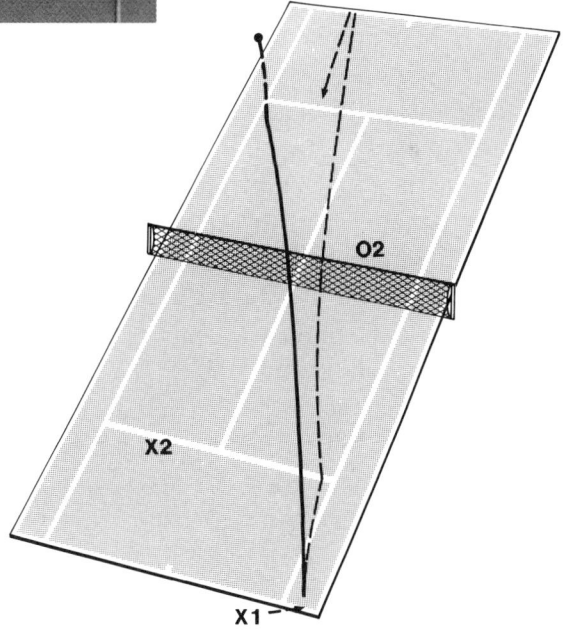

the serve is difficult to handle, think of lifting a lob over the net player.

Often, the server will hit with lessened pace on the first serve, so take the calculated risk of standing in a bit further than usual to collect the ball early, before any spin takes the ball too far away. Also, you can catch an incoming server off-balance with a quicker return from this close-in receiving position.

THE RECEIVER'S PARTNER

The partner of the receiver often provides the point-finishing shot; i.e., the serve is made, an effective return is hit which forces the server to reply softly and, **wham!!** — the receiver's partner is there to smack it away.

To play this role means being near the net at the start of the point where you will cut off half the target area for your opponents. Position yourself where you can cover your partner's typical return. If your partner usually hits pacing, low returns, be up at the net. If your partner's returns are unpredictable, hang out near the service line. And if your partner has trouble handling the serves, it will be healthier to be in the backcourt.

However, when you have a capable receiver as a partner, take up a station inside the service line. When the serve is on its way, take a quick glance back to see your partner's return. Then, shift your attention to the opponents to see their reactions, and be ready to move in if it appears they will play defensively, or to the side to cover more court if your partner is pulled wide by the serve.

MOVE FORWARD AT EVERY OPPORTUNITY

Having one player at the net and the other at the baseline is not the most effective way to play doubles. So at every opportunity the baseline player should try to join the partner at the net.

Go in behind your serve and on your opponent's second serve if you can. Use every shallow ball from your opponent as a chance to charge the net. Get into the forecourt sometimes even when you wouldn't in a singles match. A team of two, firmly entrenched at the net, presents a nearly impassable wall, with a wider arc of angles to aim for and more chances to crush away any errant lobs. The net is where doubles points are **won**.

Think **forward** before every point. Seize every chance to move up. If both of you are in the backcourt, try to make every shot a potential approach shot, and when your partner hits a return, hop forward, step forward, or lean forward — anything forward.

EXPLOIT THE MIDDLE

The alley will tempt you into hitting low percentage shots. But your opponents will often be subconsciously overprotective of the alleys, and as a result may be more vulnerable up the middle. Save the angled shots for when you're at the net. When you hit from deep in your own court, play the ball up the middle where the opposition will have less chance to send back an angled cross-court return, and the two of them may hesitate a fatal moment deciding who will take the ball.

Conversely, who should take a ball that comes back between you and your partner? There are two rules: (1) whoever is closer to the net has priority, otherwise (2) it should be the player who can hit the strongest return. If you're both at the baseline the strongest shot will probably come from whoever can hit with a forehand, but when you're both at the net it's the player who can best get the racket on the ball.

THE INFLUENCE OF LOBS

When both opponents are at the net and your team is at the baseline, take the high road. Lob often. Push your opponents away from the net and take it yourselves.

Lob early in a match to show aggressive, net-swarming opponents that you intend to keep them on the defensive. Hit the ball over the player on your right so that if that player's partner comes around to collect the ball, it will need to be hit with a backhand.

In turn, if both of you are at the net and a lob flies over your heads, both of you should retreat together. Whichever player feels they have the best play on the ball should call for it. Usually this is the partner who can get into position to return the ball from the forehand side. If it's a well-hit offensive lob you're chasing down, answer with a lob of your own. Don't bother to look where your opponents are. They probably will have come up to the net, but even if they haven't, send back a helium ball that's high enough to give the two of you time to recover for the continuation of the point.

Doubles teams should usually try to maintain a side-to-side relationship, thus when both partners are at the baseline and the opponents are at the net, a lob hit over the net players should be followed by both partners advancing to the net, as this illustration shows.

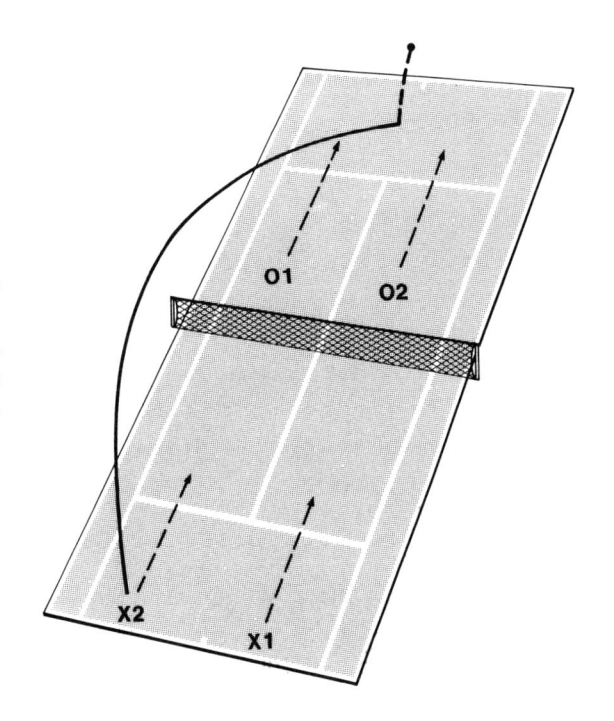

114   Tennis for Experienced Players

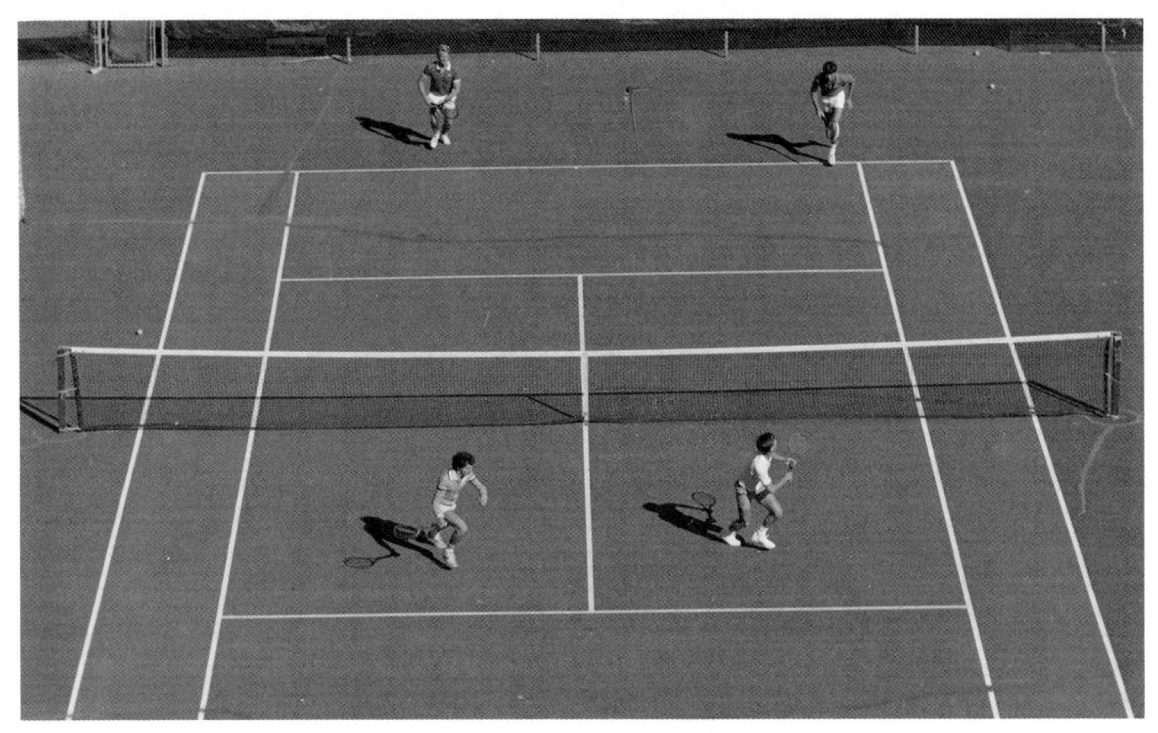

In this photo the far team has just hit an offensive lob and now begins to approach the net, while both partners of the near team retreat toward the baseline. Whoever can best get positioned to hit from the forehand side should be the player who hits the next return.

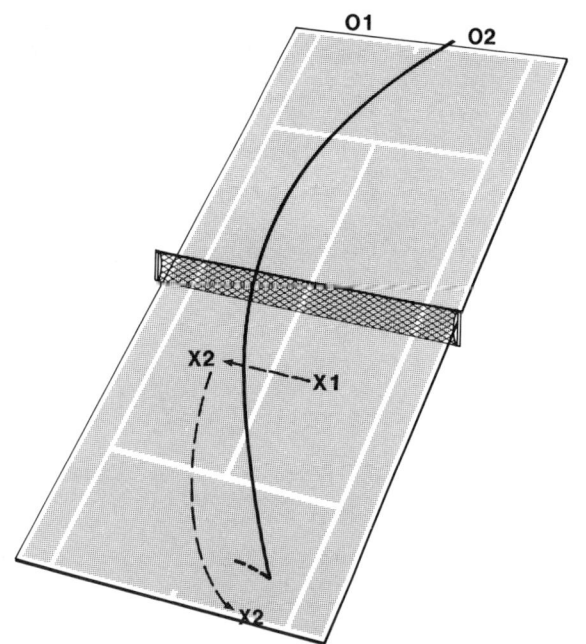

There's an exception to the side-to-side rule. This illustration shows a lob hit over the head of player X1, but high enough to allow player X2 to retreat and hit a forehand smash, thus player X1 maintains the offensive net position by crossing over to cover the area at the net vacated by X2.

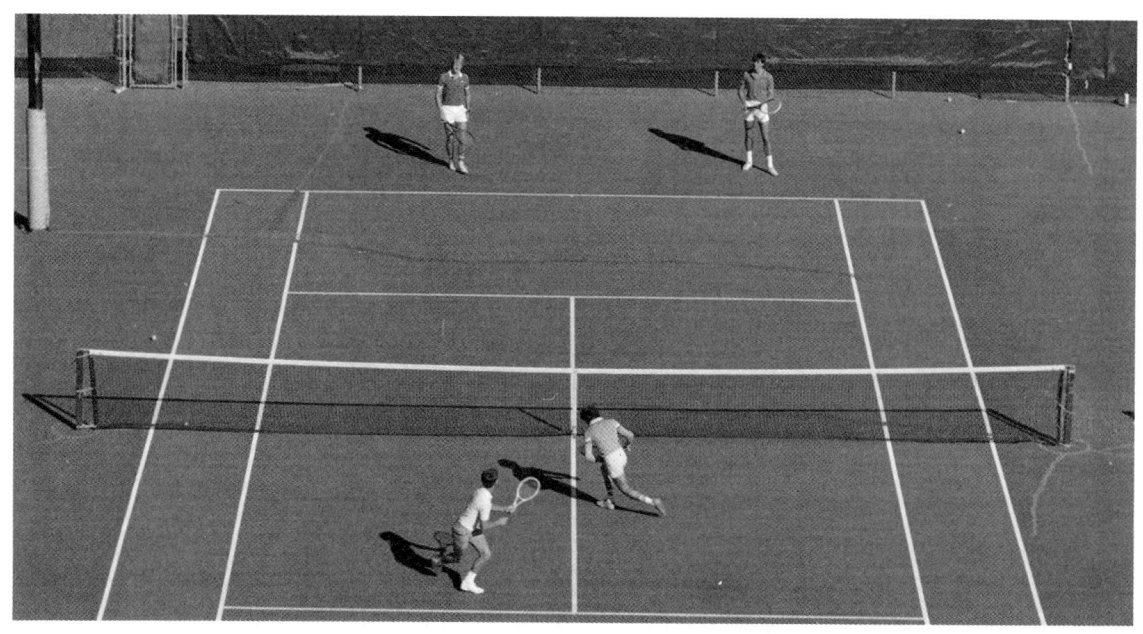

This photo shows the start of the "scissors" maneuver as the player on the left swings around the partner to prepare for a forehand smash while the player on the right stays at the net but moves over to cover the empty space. In this case, the team that hit the too-shallow lob should not approach the net. A smash return would be less likely if the lob were hit over the player on the left.

COVER THE EMPTY SPACE

Use an imaginary rope, tied between you and your partner. If your partner is forced off the side of the court, let the rope pull you over to cover the now-wider area for a return that is presented to your opponents. Always try to stay in the middle of the court space that's left over when your teammate is pushed out of position.

When one partner is pulled off the side of the court, the other partner should drift over to that side, always trying to be in the middle of the now-expanded open court space.

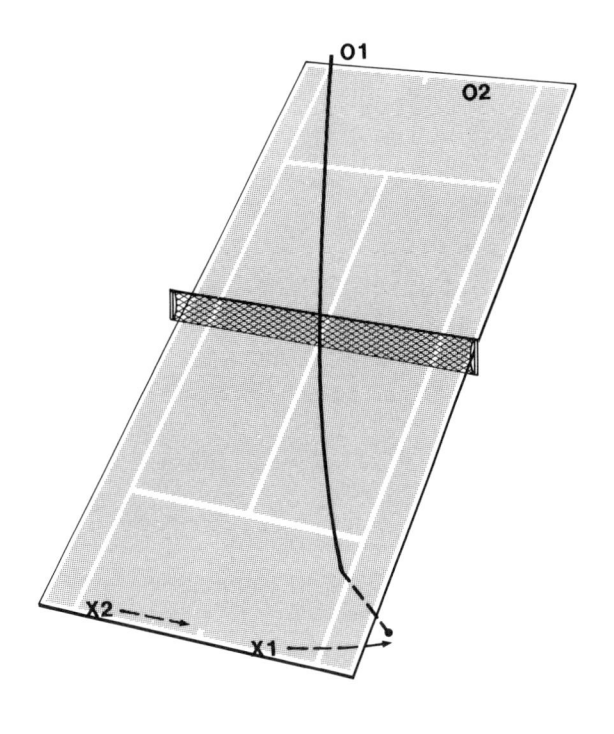

TRY AN AUSTRALIAN SERVING FORMATION

Give variety to your doubles game by sometimes using an **Australian formation** for the service. This is where the partner of the server takes a station in the same half of the court as the server, thus being directly in front of the server. Why try such an act? As a surprise for the opponents. Or just for the novelty of it. But it also presents some intriguing poaching possibilities, and when the serve is hit wide it leaves the serving team with excellent coverage to guard against a cross-court return, consequently most serves should go to the far corners instead of up-the-middle where the receiving team has a better chance to attack the flanks of the serving team.

The Australian formation is especially effective when the server hits into the far corner of the ad court. It's a virtual guarantee that the next shot for the serving team will be a forehand (off a presumably weak return as a bonus).

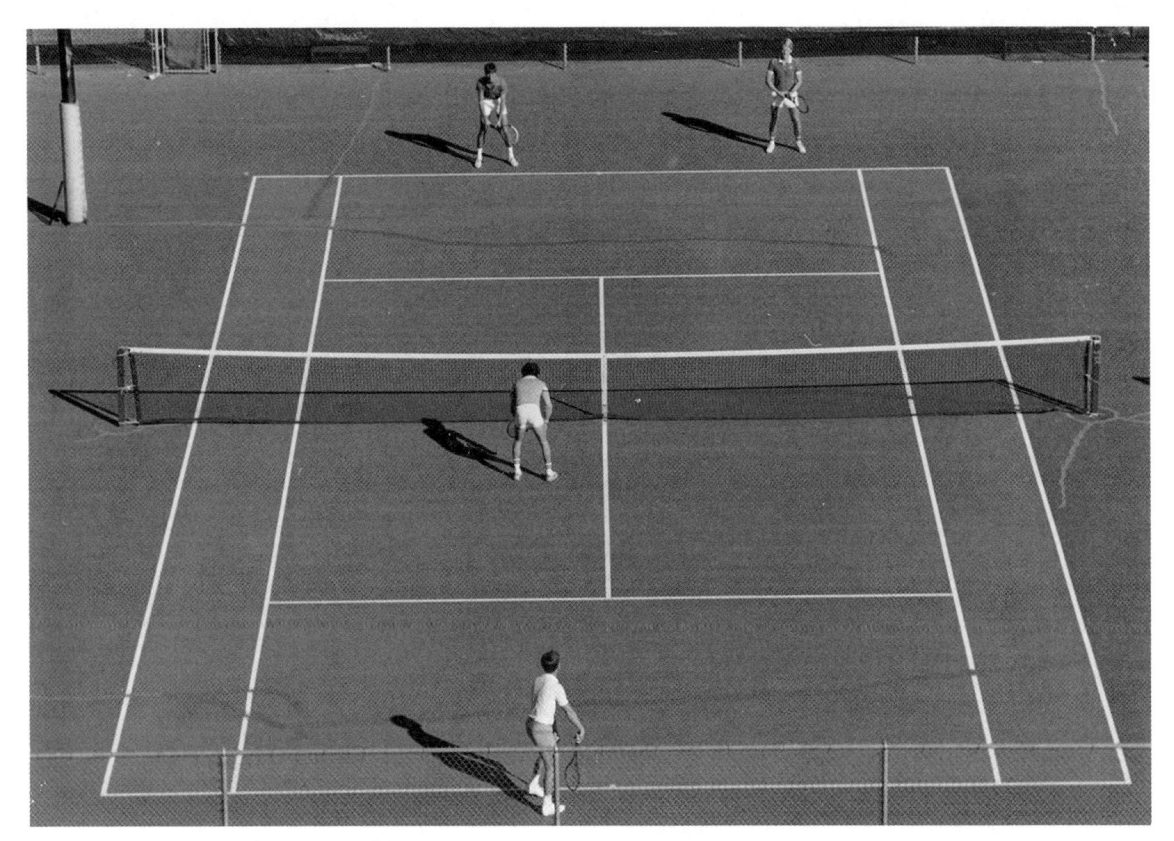

Here's the start of the Australian formation for serving into the ad court, where both the server and the server's partner are on the same half of their court. Note that the server stands near the center mark. If the serve is hit to the far corner, the serving team is almost assured the return will come to their forehand sides.

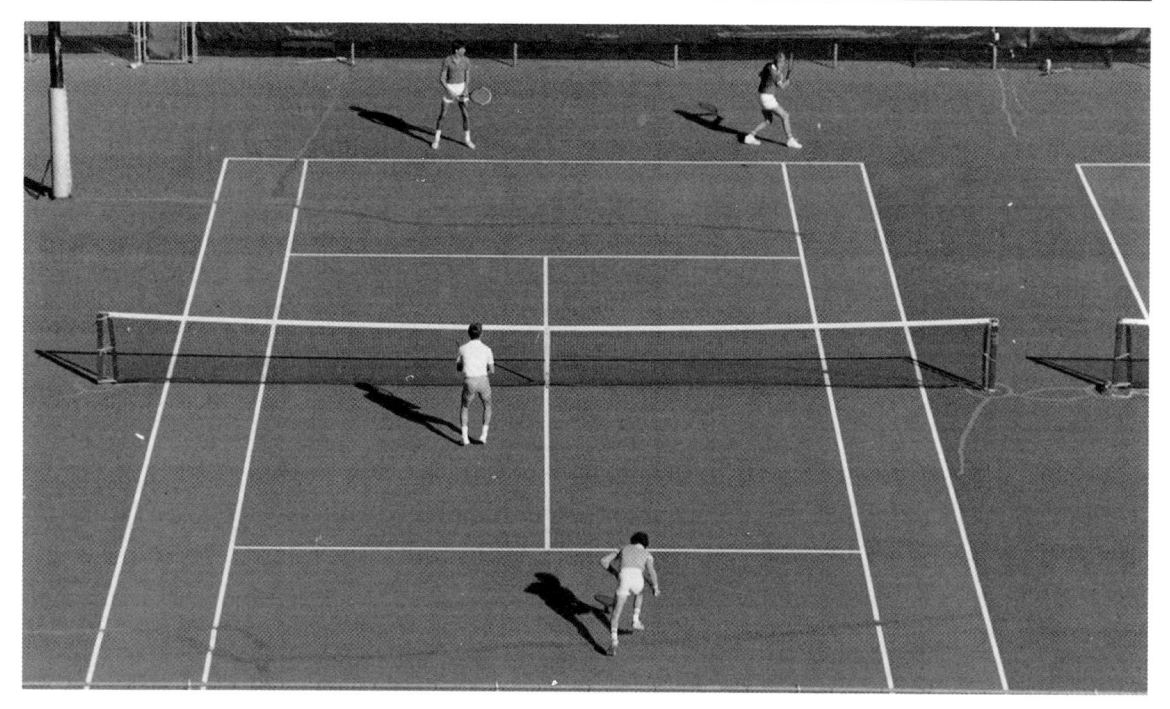

Here the server has done the proper job, from the Australian formation, of sending the ball to the far corner. If the server then charges the net the run should be on a diagonal, following along the path of the ball, rather than straight forward.

MIXED DOUBLES

Add this to the long list of credits for tennis: it's one of the few sports where men and women compete as teammates, against other mixed teams, including at the professional level.

Mixed doubles is what you make it. It can be friendly socializing through a game, or a refreshing diversion, or darned good tennis. Above all, it's like any other doubles: four people enjoying tennis instead of two.

The criteria of play for mixed doubles is the same as for any other doubles match: the most capable partner serves first, and the most dependable partner should receive serve in the ad court. There are no special rules, and no special provisions. So the timeworn inquiry of "Tennis, anyone?" could be paraphrased into "Tennis is for everyone." It's for both sexes, and all ages, at the same time, any time.

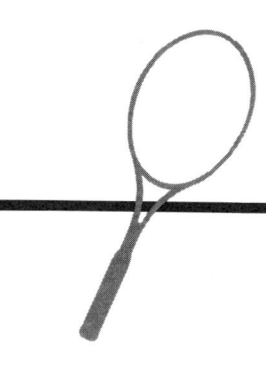

Chapter Ten

How To Be Mentally Tough

It's predictable. When you're playing well everything is in sync; mind and body together. The ball is as big as a grapefruit and seems to be coming in slow motion. Your swing has infinite harmony and every shot finds its mark.

Yet at other times, you can be in total disillusion with your play. You get caught frozen between points, your shots have no life, and the ball is erratic. Play poorly, and you feel terrible.

But — usually you play poorly **because** you feel terrible. Negative states of mind can be devastating to your game. If you're nervous, frustrated, angry — your play will be fitful. But if you're alive, energetic, confident — your shots will have vivid resolution.

The proper mental and emotional states will help you to mobilize the energy sources that are crucial for optimal performance. So before each match, generate positive attitudes. Forge an upbeat emotional tone that will transfer into rousing play. Talk yourself into an optimistic frame of reference. Convince yourself that all will go well.

HANDLING STRESS BEFORE A MATCH

You've entered a tournament and you thought it was going to be fun until match time, when anxiety begins to take over. You're not alone, because **everyone** is nervous before an important match, including the pros and including your opponent. If you are often too keyed up before competition, try the following:

1. **Think constructively.** If your apprehensive mind starts to build a series of potential reasons why you might not play well, think instead of the things you will be able to **do** during the match. Focus on the skills you know you already have. Visually picture them. See yourself doing well. There's only a given amount of thinking space in your brain, so if you fill it with constructive thoughts they will crowd out the negative ones.
2. **Be honest with yourself.** Realize that there is, after all, only so much you can do in the match. There's no way to make last-minute changes in your ability. You are what you are — nothing more, nothing less.
3. **Bring enough equipment.** Two rackets are a must, as insurance for a broken string. The spare racket should be one you've played with before. Also, bring new tennis balls, a towel, water, hat, and even extra shoestrings.
4. **Be on time.** But not too early. If you must wait a long time before the match, tension might multiply. If you're on time but your match is delayed, don't intently watch any ongoing matches.
5. **Find a place to relax.** If you're reasonably calm, just sit or lie down to take the weight off your feet. But if you're really uptight and can't relax passively, then do something active — walk around, do some stretching exercises, or even jog a bit.
6. **Be physically ready.** Avoid any unnecessary drains of your strength on game day. Consume high-carbohydrate calories the night before, and have your last full meal at least four hours before match time.
7. **Treat it as a game.** In the final analysis, competitive play should add **enjoyment** to your life, not frustration. It's a game, the purpose of which is to reduce stress, not create it. No matter how well or poorly you play, after it's over everything will still be intact. You'll still have your job, your college credits, your wallet, your stamp collection, your friends, and your own psyche.

WHAT TO DO DURING THE WARM-UP

Use the pre-match warm-up time to alert all your resources — organize both mind and muscles. Create the right state of mental and physical readiness.

1. **Actually warm-up.** Get your body temperature elevated. Do little hops between your practice shots. Stretch your limbs out, giving flexibility to your muscles. Be **physically ready** to go all out on the first point of the first game. Be ready to assume the offensive at the very start.
2. **Prepare all your strokes.** Practice every one of your strokes, not only forehands and backhands, but also volleys, overheads, and lobs. In particular, make sure you have hit plenty of serves. Hit your shots easily at first, then with increasing pace. Try especially to sense the rhythm of

your swing. Remind your muscles of how it feels to hit with the fluid freedom that comes so easily during a practice session.

3. **Create positive energy.** Channel your supercharged state into positive form. As soon as you walk onto the court, start working immediately to collect confident energy. Feel alive. Be optimistic. Sense the very thrill of being able to play. Create electricity in your muscles. Grab hold of your inner self and mesmerize yourself with positive self-talk.

4. **Nothing fancy.** Make up your mind that you are going to play with the talent you have, not trying anything you haven't yet acquired in your hitting repertoire. No whimsical attempts at, for example, top-spin lobs if you haven't mastered a topspin lob.

5. **Evaluate your opponent.** Take an inventory of your rival. Notice if there is a weaker groundstroke side. Offer varieties of pace to see the response. Get your opponent up to the net to observe talent and aggressiveness.

6. **Center on yourself.** Do not be affected before the match begins by things that have no relationship to the contest. If your opponent is wearing designer attire and has expensive equipment, this could be intimidating. Or your rival's court behavior might be irksome. Perhaps it seems your adversary isn't taking you seriously enough. Remember that the major objective of the warm-up is to get **yourself** ready, not to become obsessed with the characteristics of your opposition. This is **your** time. Use this important moment to focus attention on the rhythm and timing of your own strokes. Alert your muscles to the job you have for them. Become self-centered.

WHEN THE MATCH BEGINS

One factor that consistently emerges as a common trait among top-level athletes in any sport is an ability to focus attention on what is relevant to their performance. They are able to block out extraneous stimuli and concentrate on their task. They use selective attention — being alert to what is meaningful and ignoring the rest. They focus on their strokes, not on the wind, the sun, the prize, the spectators, nor anything else.

Do the same — selectively attend to the match. It isn't meaningful, for example, to think of your overdue rent, or the unfinished term paper, or the problem with your car, or the distractions on the neighboring court. Extraneous stimuli must get ruled out — tennis in.

EACH POINT IS AN ENTITY

It's vital to selectively attend not only to the match as a whole, but also to isolate on each point — in fact on each **ball**. Hone your attention on every shot. Don't be affected by your performance in a previous game, or a previous point, or even the last ball of an ongoing exchange. Tunnel into every ball.

If you hit a poor shot, put it out of your mind and instantly self-talk confidence back into your attitude. Between points, loosen your muscles, take the racket out of your hitting hand, and bounce a few times on your toes. You'll recover your alertness and positive frame of mind more quickly by relaxing than by fighting yourself after an errant shot. Be ready to hit rhythmically again, on the next ball.

Try this technique: play every point as if it were the deciding one in a game. That way you'll focus on one point at a time, and collectively it will add up to a higher level of concentration for the whole match.

Make sure that you're ready for the start of every point. If you're serving, bounce the ball a few times to gather your emotions, fix in your mind where you want the ball to go, then **sense** the spin and pace you will give to the ball. If you're receiving, try to build your focus in coordination with your opponent's serve. Endow your muscles with a feeling of fluid readiness, perhaps doing a few hops to help the feeling. As your opponent bounces the ball, begin to collect your alertness. See the server as a whole, but when the toss is made, zero in on the ball, like a zoom lens, to where you have a heightened visual clarity when the ball is on its way.

STAY UNDER CONTROL

Sometimes you just can't help it. As a match progresses, frustration over mistakes or growing nervousness takes over. Although your head knows better, your emotions won't let your arms and legs respond. So acknowledge that you're getting rattled. Combat the feeling by taking more time between points. Relax your grip, shrug your shoulders, shake out your legs. Take at least one deep breath before the start of the next point, and visualize what you want to do with that point. Stay ritualistic. Stick to your routines between points to provide yourself with something familiar and therefore reassuring.

Remember that your body responds to your mental attitudes. Tell it positive things. Believe that you are capable. Then hit your backhands freely. Belt your serves with conviction. Hit your volleys with confidence. Tell yourself how good you feel, and your nerve-muscle machinery will respond.

PLAY POSITIVE TENNIS

When you are optimistic, believing in your own ability, then you can play **positive tennis**. It means trying to win points rather than trying to avoid **losing** them.

There's a difference in style. The player who tries mostly to avoid making mistakes will hit cautiously, conservatively, without spontaneity. The backswing becomes shorter, there is less acceleration in the swing, and the serve is tentative. Even the body language changes: slumped shoulders, lowered head, nervous fidgeting.

By contrast, the player who wants to **win points** will hit with affirmative, free-swinging strokes. They finish every swing. They do not hold back on the serve. They **punish** the ball!

Both players will make mistakes. However, the player who hits to avoid errors will make **negative** mistakes: dumping the ball into the net, hitting too shallow, pushing the second serve. But the player who hits to win will make **positive** mistakes: the ball will be hit too long rather than too short; they'll try for an ace on the second serve; they'll come up to the net at the wrong time. It's because they are trying to **make things happen.** Positive mistakes are part of energetic, optimistic play. They indicate you are playing with freedom in your style, and probably even that you are enjoying the game more.

BELIEVE THAT YOUR SERVE WILL GO IN

Arnold Palmer, golfer extraordinaire, once said that when he hit a perfect shot he was never surprised, since that's what he **wanted** to do. He was only surprised, he said, when the ball did **not** go where he wanted.

Serving is no different. If you anticipate failure, you'll never be surprised when you double fault. And getting the first serve in may be cause for astonishment.

It's another example of negative tennis. Instead, believe that **every** serve will go in. To facilitate such a mindset, walk slowly to your serving station, then take only one ball in your hand for the first serve — stick the second one in your pocket. Collect yourself both mentally and physically before starting the motion. Have all your decisions made: where to hit the ball, with how much pace, how much spin, and what you will do after the serve. Physically "feel" your swing and mentally "see" the ball go in, even before you make the toss. Then just let your body act out the mental image that you have created for it. You'll hit more serves in, and not one of them will be a surprise.

ACT LIKE A WINNER

No matter how you happen to be playing at the moment, act like a winner, even if it's an **act**. The way you behave **physically** will transfer to how you **feel.**

Watch a champion. There is confidence in every manner — the way they approach the line to serve, the way they flaunt their playing talents, even defiant amazement at losing a point. A winner is dauntless, animated, lively. By contrast, an unsure player will walk around the court two inches shorter than they actually are. The whole body droops, and confidence stays down with it.

So be **tall.** Put assurance in your style. If you're nervous, shake out you shoulders and settle your tension. Slow down and be deliberate. Have a controlled, affirmative air to your behavior. Use your physical self to persuade your mental self that you are capable and ready to play well.

CLOSE OUT YOUR OPPONENT

Sometimes, if you build a lead in a match and then allow your intensity to slacken, it may be difficult to regain the edge later in the match if your opponent makes a comeback. This is likely to happen, in particular, right after having broken your opponent's serve. You might feel that you've accomplished an end in itself, and now you can relax somewhat. But if in turn you lose your own serve, your rival may be rejuvenated.

Other signs of a loss of competitive instinct are: easing up on the serve, turning conservative with shot placement, not hitting to an opponent's weaker side, and not coming up to the net. Worst of all, the efficiency of stroke production may begin to falter.

There **are** times when you're in full control of a match and it becomes difficult to maintain a high level of focused attention. But in these cases a subtle "easing off" will go unnoticed by your (not wanting to be embarrassed) opponent, and you can concentrate more on the rhythm of your strokes instead of trying to drive the ball with power. Use your second serve to start points, or attend more to your footwork, and practice the useful art of hitting the ball deep up the middle. But when you have an opponent on the ropes, and victory is imminent, then finish your work.

IF YOU'RE LOSING

Get control of yourself. Maintain your cool. Use self-talk to stay relaxed. When you fall behind in a match, there is a tendency to tighten up, to abbreviate your strokes, and to play defensively. So exaggerate your relaxation routines. Consciously ease your grip. Take the racket out of your hitting hand between points. Take more deep breaths. Bounce more on your toes.

Take time between games to analyze both your game and that of your opponent. If you are beating yourself with errors, concentrate more on rhythm and on watching the ball. If your opponent is winning with power, change the pace of your shots. If you haven't been coming up to the net, try that. But do not press yourself into suddenly trying exotic shots you haven't mastered. Don't try what you can't do. Only make the changes you are capable of executing. Keep the basic fundamental of strategy in mind: know what you do best, figure out what your opponent does worst, and link the two together.

TALK TO YOURSELF

Your body is listening. How you feel affects how you play, and you'll play your best when you are calm and confident. Tennis is a difficult game to play when you are too emotional. Your body doesn't respond. Your head knows what to do but your obstinate arms and legs won't listen.

Is it possible to talk yourself into relaxing? Of course it is. You can substantially reduce your feelings of nervousness and frustration by positive self-conversation. Put on your own headset. Talk to your own brain. Commit yourself to becoming disciplined in what you say to yourself, just like you have disciplined your physical skills. If self-destructive thoughts enter your brain, interrupt them. Say **"Stop!"** Replace them with encouragements instead. Tell yourself, "O.K., I hit a lousy shot. But forget it. Keep scrambling. This next point is mine!"

It's normal to berate yourself after a poor shot. But then switch mental gears. Self-talk your brain into a confident readiness for the next point. As you feel, so you are.

GO SEE THE MOVIE IN YOUR HEAD

The most widely used mental enhancement technique in sports incorporates the mind's lucid capacity for imagination. Through a technique of visual dramatization called **mental practice**, an athlete will, while in a state of quietude, create a mental image of their own performance, trying in the process to generate all the sensations and environmental conditions of the skill, including the actual feel of the execution. It is a virtual dreamland of rehearsal, and it grows more powerful in effect as a person gains in experience.

The best results occur when you are in a quiet, nondistracting environment and your mind is not cluttered with thoughts or feelings unrelated to the sport. There are two ways to use visualization. One is to see yourself performing as if you were an observer — a spectator watching your own game. The other is to stay inside yourself, seeing the events of a tennis match as you would with your own eyes when actually playing. Research suggests that the second of the two may be more beneficial for those with extensive playing experience.

Following is a general guideline for using mental practice:

1. Choose a time and place where you can be undisturbed.
2. Close your eyes, breathe deeply, and relax as completely as possible. Feel your muscles go limp.
3. Clear your mind. Imagine a blank screen. Think of emptiness. Free your mind of all thoughts.
4. Select an aspect of tennis — serve, forehand, whatever. Visualize yourself performing the skill, including all parts of the execution. For example, if you rehearse the serve, see yourself stepping up to the line, bouncing the ball, setting your sights, and so on, right through the end result of the landing and rebound of the served ball.
5. Visualize your performance in as much detail as possible.
6. Visualize in color, making the colors as vivid as you can. For example, emphasize the contrast between the color of the ball and the sky or the playing surface.
7. Try to **feel** the movements of the game. Create the very physical sensations of the performance.
8. Mentally practice with all your senses. Not only should you see and feel the skills of the game, you should also **hear** the sounds of tennis, such as the thwack of the ball, even distracting noises like passing traffic or chatter from a neighboring court.
9. Rehearse the emotions of tennis, especially sensing yourself in full command of your psyche during stressful points in a match.
10. Sometimes visualize in slow motion, trying to be critically analytical of your skill during these slowed-down performances.
11. Give some time to freewheeling imaginations, allowing spontaneous visualizations to arise of, for example, a rousing exchange of strong shots between you and your opponent.
12. End each session by seeing yourself hitting some emphatic, convincing, point-winning shots.
13. Don't prolong the mental practice. Several brief sessions of five minutes or so are better than one long session.
14. Gradually try to incorporate mental practice into your on-court playing so you can use quick visual reminders between points, or during an exchange of sides, or before a serve.

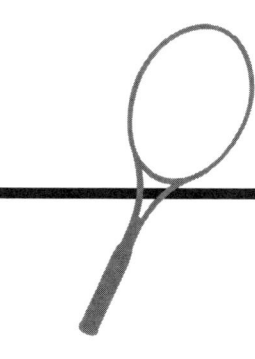

Chapter Eleven

Realistic Practice

Practice makes perfect, it's commonly said. There are also other myths about athletic skills.

Practice alone does not make perfect — it merely makes more **permanent** the things that are practiced. It's possible to practice the **wrong** things, thereby making **flaws** in performance more permanent. Every time a swing is executed the nervous system remembers, to some extent, until it's a habit. And habit is practice long pursued until it's difficult to do it any other way.

So do well during practice sessions. Teach your nervous system to remember only its very best.

MAKE PRACTICE LIKE THE GAME

Any practice session should be realistic. It should simulate the actual game, or small segments of the game, so that it's more "real-life" than merely hitting the ball incessantly back and forth without purpose. Creating game-like circumstances makes practice more interesting and gives reason to do well.

For example, if you're uncertain about your play at the net, instead of starting a practice point with a serve, start instead by hitting a groundstroke, and have your practice partner feed you a half-speed shallow ball which allows you to come in to hit an approach shot. After that, play the point out as normal.

Or, say you have trouble returning serves. Have your partner hit off-speed serves to you, and each time you get the return back between the service line and baseline you score a point.

Have difficulty handling pressure in a match? You can get better by introducing some pressure into these game rehearsals. For instance, you could play "one serve" points where you get only one chance to make the serve good. Or you could reduce the court by agreeing that any ball which lands in front of the service line will be called out. Or you could play an entire set of tie-breaker games.

Pick out your weakest, or least confident aspects of the game, and create situations that will help you develop the necessary skills. Put aside any insecurities. For example, if your backhand is a troublesome area, you might play some points where only backhands are allowed. Remember that the more advanced you become in this game, the more your weaker areas will be exploited by opponents. So devote plenty of practice time to fixing any inadequate parts of your play. And don't overlook such often-neglected aspects as second serves, half-volleys, and drop shots.

CREATING MUSCLE MEMORY

If there is no structure at all to practice it's too easy to slip into lethargic habits such as not bending the knees, or failing to transfer the weight properly, or letting the racket be lazy. Purposeless hitting of the ball is an invitation to making flaws habitual.

In effect, each time a ball is hit there is a neural pathway electrochemically set off that becomes more and more permanent every time the same pattern is used. Then, in the future, any similar situation (as in a game) will kick into action the same neural pathways that had been ingrained during practice. Consequently, it's important to develop a "muscle memory" in practice which is correct in technique and easily transferable to match play.

Try especially to instill a muscle memory for a big put-away shot. For example, if you have good control of a cross-court topspin forehand, then hit it every chance you get in practice. Implant the pattern so deep into your nervous system that each time the opportunity to hit the shot in a match arises, all you need to do is pull the switch and: **click!** — another topspin cross-court winner!

REHEARSE BOTH OFFENSE AND DEFENSE

It's natural in practice to focus on offensive shots. But defense should not be overlooked. For instance, it's unlikely that attention will be given to retrieving a lob while on the run away from the net, or intentionally hitting from just behind the service line, or even service returns. A complete practice should have both offensive and defensive shot rehearsal.

In a match the offensive intent is to hit the ball with enough pace and/or placement to either win the point outright or to force a weak return. Offensive tennis, therefore, is built around the following:

1. Hitting the ball into the corners.
2. Hitting overpowering serves.
3. Coming to the net behind a strong serve or a well-placed approach shot.
4. Hitting offensive lobs.
5. Hitting the ball out of the opponent's reach.

On defense, the objective is to stay alive in a point; to play the ball in a way that will keep the opponent from hitting the next shot for a winner. Thus, in a match you would:

1. Hit a defensive lob.
2. Retrieve a ball while on the run.
3. Return strong serves.
4. Stretch for a wide volley at the net.
5. Respond to any defensive predicament with a return hit deep up the middle.

Basically, in a tennis match you either (1) make things happen, or you must (2) respond to things that happen. Practice sessions often ignore the second of the two. But the staged rehearsal of an offensive shot by one partner will usually present an opportunity for the other partner to practice defensive returns of that shot.

For example, one player might hit aggressive topspin groundstrokes, while the other tries to loft the ball back with off-speed returns. In this way one player gets tuned for crunching a slow-moving ball for a winner, while the other can rehearse the change-of-pace shots that are useful in a match against a big hitter.

A SUGGESTED PRACTICE SESSION

There are no ultimate practice routines. The major objectives are quite simply to:

1. Have a partner who is willing to **practice** instead of just wanting to play matches.
2. Rehearse the things that will **actually happen** in a match.
3. Make the sessions **enjoyable.**

Accordingly, a typical day of practice might be organized as follows:

1. **Warm up** properly, including stretching, before hitting.
2. **Hit easily** for the first few minutes, using only groundstrokes. Have no target other than keeping the ball within reach of your partner. Concentrate on the form of the strokes and the rhythm of your swing.
3. Now give your shots more **dimension**. For instance, try to land every ball within a yard of the baseline. Or try hitting a "heavy" ball by emphasizing the acceleration of the racket head.
4. Next, try some **placement** hitting, where you aim your shots toward a specific area of the court. For example, hit only cross-court with your partner, corner to corner, and gradually increase the intensity of this drill.
5. Now play **rapid fire**, where both of you stand across the net from each other, just inside the service line, and hit volley after volley, trying to keep the ball in play as long as possible.
6. Then it's **setup time,** where your partner

feeds you exactly the shot you want. Often this is best accomplished if your partner hits a bucket of balls to you, without attempting to return your shots.

7. Add **serve** and **receive** practice. Hit half-a-bucket while your partner hits returns. No playing points out — just concentrate on serves and returns. Then switch roles.
8. Now for some **match play** drills. Try to stage actual playing situations. Be inventive with these drills, but don't overcomplicate them. Make the situations as close to reality as possible. This part of the practice may be the longest, and the most profitable.
9. Devote time to **specialty shots**, such as drop shots, topspin lobs, or backhand overheads. Give attention to the shots you'll be forced to hit defensively in a match.
10. Finish off the day with **free hitting**, focusing again on rhythm and form. That'll get you in the right frame of mind to feel good about the day, and in a positive reference for the next match.

JUST FOR THE FUN OF IT

There's always the potential of losing sight of the purpose of tennis. It's to enjoy playing — to have pure, unadulterated fun. This is, after all, a **game**.

Practice should be invigorating. If it's drudgery, little benefit will emerge. There may even be some negative outcomes.

Make practice fun. Add variety to the sessions. Use the time to experiment with different spins, or new ways to hit the ball. Even be crazy sometimes by doing such things as hitting the ball with the racket in your non-preferred hand. Or play some points where there is no limit on the number of times the ball can bounce before being returned. Or agree that after every shot you must touch the service line with your racket.

Let these whimsical little games be totally therapeutic. Use them to spark renewed interest in practice. In the bargain you'll be reminded that tennis is a sporting endeavor, the end result of which should be, above all else, to add enjoyment to your life.

AN AEROBIC WORKOUT

Practice sessions can be arranged to incorporate both a rehearsal of skills and aerobic conditioning. In this way your body will become accustomed to hitting polished shots while being pressed into a high level of energy output. It's also a fun way of adding variety and dimension to practice.

You can readily design your own aerobic workout, focusing in particular on the parts of the game that you want to practice the most. The eight drills given on the following pages are offered as an example.

Four-Ball Rally. (Not illustrated) Each player gets two balls ready. One player starts a point by hitting a second serve, just to get the point underway. As soon as a winner is hit or an error is made, the second player hits a new ball into play, within the other player's reach, and the point continues until all four balls have been played.

Corner Rally.
Both players run from corner to corner. Player A hits only down-the-line shots, while player B hits only cross-court shots. When a winner or error is produced, another ball is immediately put into play so the rhythm of the exchange is not broken. After awhile, hitting roles exchange.

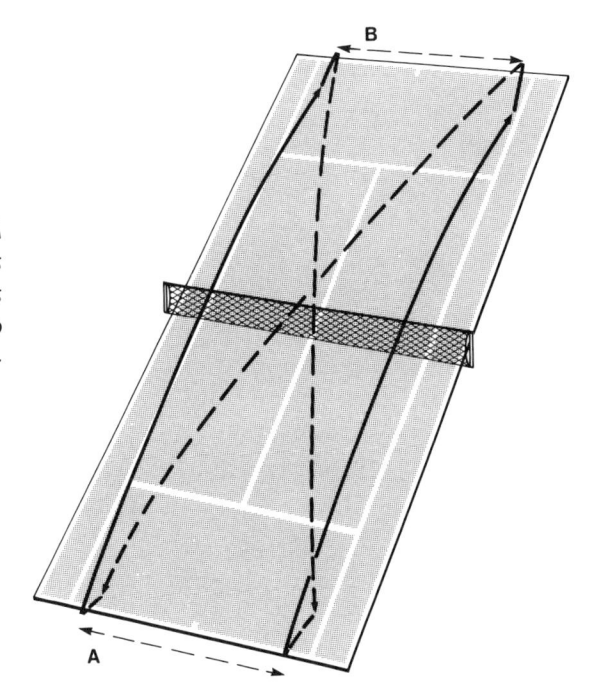

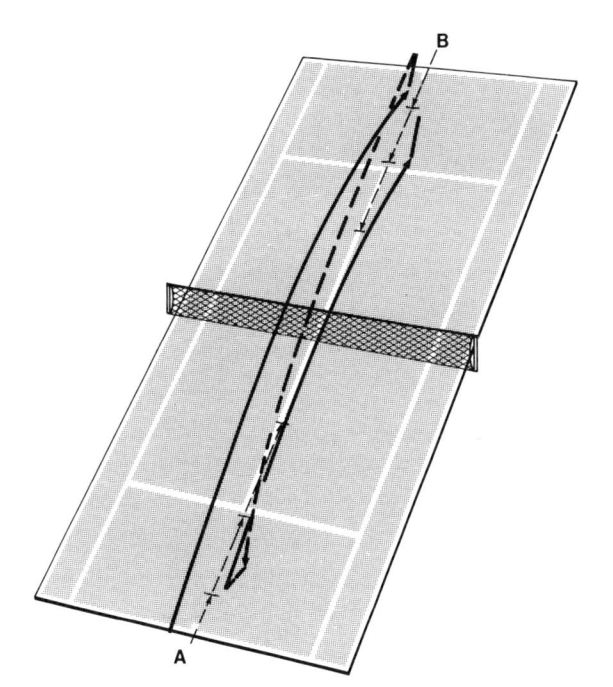

Hit-and-advance.
Both players start from behind the baseline, each carrying two or three balls ready for play. A groundstroke starts the rally, each player advancing toward the net after every shot. If a ball is misplayed, another is immediately put into play. Eventually, both players are across the net from each other, playing rapid-fire volleys.

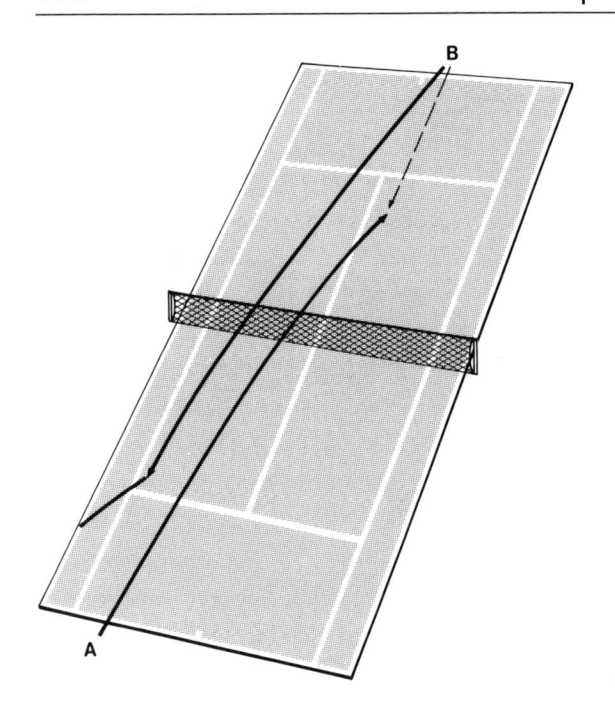

Serve-and-Volley.
Player B serves and advances toward the net. Player A does not attempt to return the serve, but hits a ready ball to player B, who plays a volley, and the point is then played to its finish. As a variation, player A could have another ball ready to provide a lob after player B has hit the volley. After the point, roles switch.

Machine-Gun Volleys.
Player B has bucket of balls and hits one after the other in rapid succession to player A, who scrambles to return them from a station at the net. Player B varies the pace and placement of each ball, and player A must try to volley every one. Switch roles with player A is exhausted.

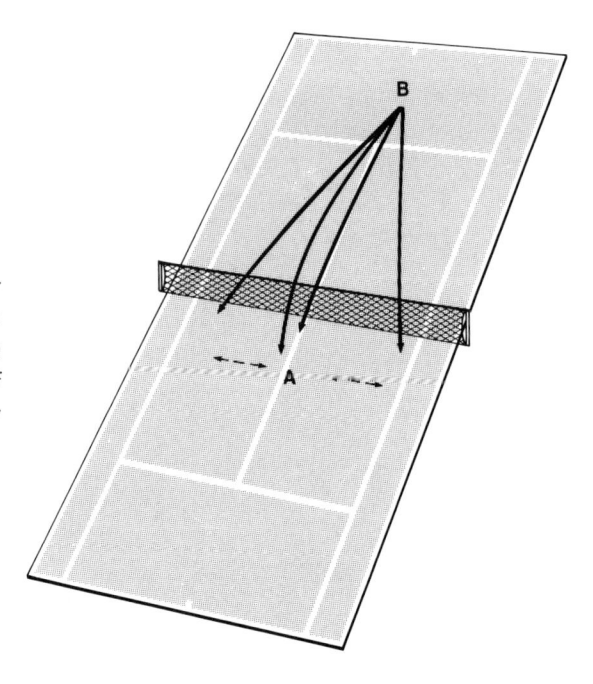

All-Court Scramble.
Player B has a bucket of balls, and hits a variety of placements to any part of the court. Player A tries to chase down and return every ball. Player B keeps up the feed of balls, nonstop, until player A runs out of energy, then roles reverse.

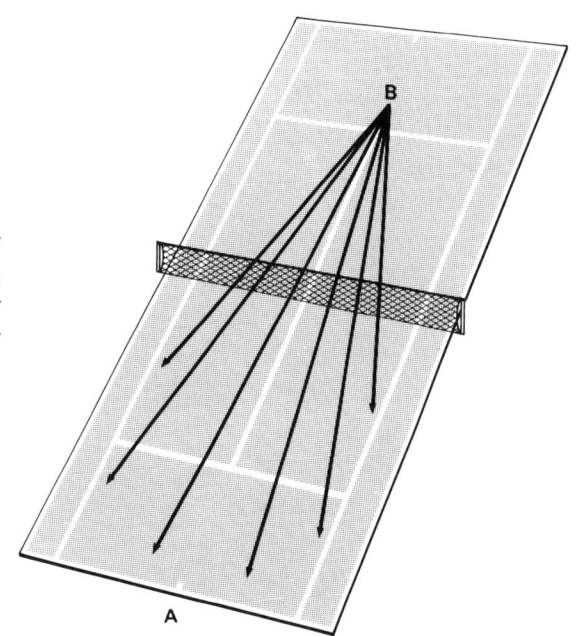

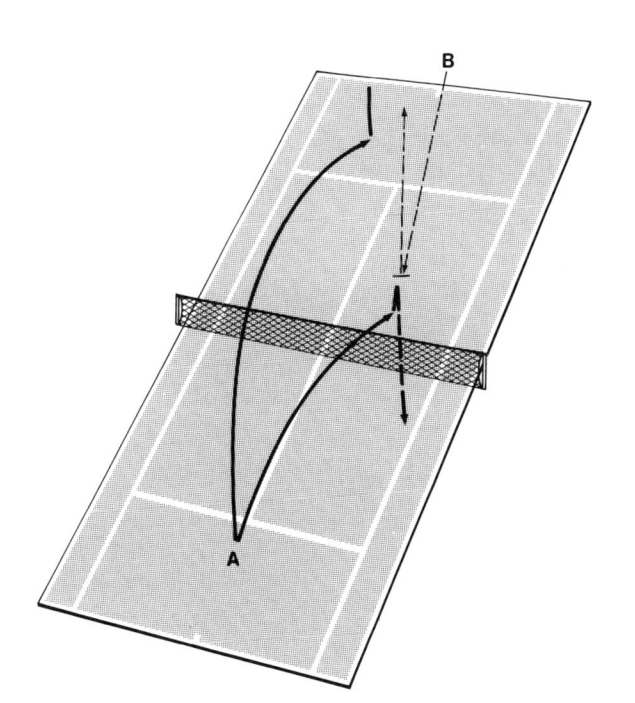

Up-and-Back.
Player A stands between the baseline and service line, with a bucket of balls, and first hits a short ball that player B must run down. Then player A follows with a lob which player B retreats to hit, and player A provides another shallow ball. Player A does not try to return any ball, but alternates hitting shallow and deep shots.

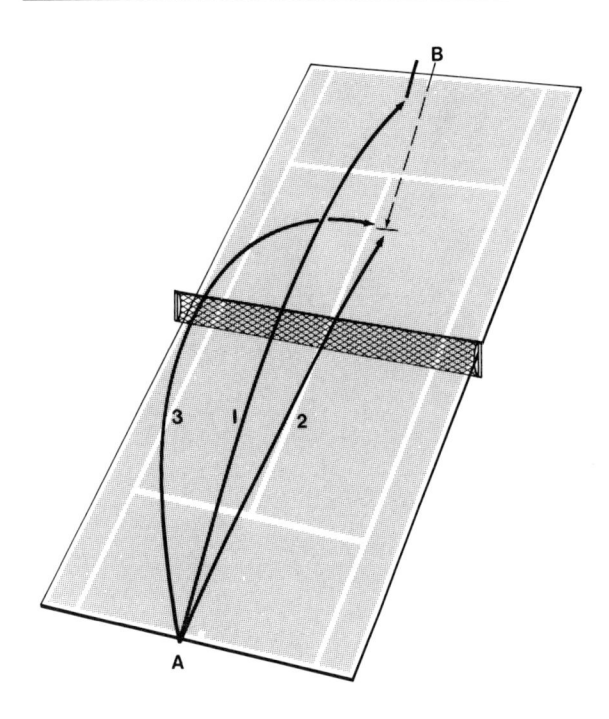

Three-Shot Sequence.
Player A has three balls ready and hits the first one to player B, who is behind the baseline. Player B hits a deep shot and advances toward the net. Player A hits the next ball to the feet of player B, who returns a half-volley and finishes the charge to the net where player A lifts up a lob for player B to smash.

Chapter Twelve

The Advantage of High-Tech Equipment

Today a player can look frighteningly good in tennis attire that is comfortable on the court and aesthetic enough to be worn at a lawn party after a match. And orthopedic shoes have eliminated the plight of skidding around the court in footwear that did not have support in all the right places. But it is the instrument of play, the racket, which must measure up to the hitting capabilities of the player.

RACKET CHARACTERISTICS

All rackets that deliver excellent playability are composites — a crossbreed of several materials. The great majority are made of graphite that is bonded with other reinforcing space-age compounds into a matrix that is lightweight and strong so you can swing faster while still maintaining control. Graphite is the best material for bonding with others, and has the most effective vibration-damping qualities to absorb the shock of the ball at impact.

Manufacturers can combine materials with racket design to produce variable degrees of racket stiffness — a critical characteristic of how much a frame will bend on impact with the ball. Stiff rackets bend less and therefore the ball loses less energy at impact to produce a higher resultant velocity in rebound. With flexible frames energy is lost as the frame yields to impact and the ball has less impulse from its rebound. However, flexible frames allow more shock-damping and cushioning — good news for players with elbow problems.

The thickness of the frame can also control stiffness, and thus the advent, in the early 1990's, of the wide-body design. By increasing the cross-section of the frame, stiffness can be increased, so as a rule the bulkier the frame the stiffer the racket. If you like to hit hard, a stiff frame may be the best choice. If you are more of a steady baseline player, a flexible racket is probably more functional.

THE PLAYABILITY OF THE RACKET

How easily a racket handles in actual play is largely determined by its size, weight, and balance point (that point where the racket would balance on a knife edge). A handle heavy racket has its balance point in the lower half of the frame, toward the handle. With more of the weight in the handle half of the racket, it will be quicker on serves and at the net. A head-heavy racket has more weight in the top half of the frame and is considered to be better for baseline play.

When they are play-tested for performance ratings, rackets are generally analyzed for (1) power, which is the potential to transfer energy to the ball, (2) control, defined as the racket's ability to direct the ball to where it's intended to be hit, (3) maneuverability, which is how easy or difficult it is to start the racket into motion and its overall mobility on all strokes, and (4) comfort, which is how it absorbs the vibration of ball impact and how much it twists on off-center hits.

When a ball is hit off-center, especially toward the sides of the racket, the frame will twist along its long axis. This twisting effect can decrease the accuracy of the shot, thus rackets can also be described relative to their "sweet spot," that being the string hitting area which provides the best power with consistent ball control, and the least shock and vibration. Generally, rackets with larger heads (100 square inches and larger), and which have greater stiffness and heavier weights will have the larger sweetspots. However, rackets with very large heads may twist too much because of their larger radius for rotation on off-center hits.

BUY INTELLECTUALLY, NOT EMOTIONALLY

Human tennis psyche too easily compels us to purchase a power-laden racket. But the ideal racket is one that maximizes both power and control. Every player has a personal point where power and control are in perfect harmony with the qualities of the racket. Buying the wrong racket will not optimize your game. So be realistic about your own playing characteristics. Find a racket that compliments your strengths. If, for example, you already hit with sufficient power, you will not necessarily do better with a stiffer, wide-body racket. There are no good rackets and bad rackets, only bad combinations of player and racket.

Just as you would seek medical advice from someone trained, go to a pro shop or tennis specialty store for advice on a new racket. They make tennis their only business. Borrow a "demo" and take it out on the court. Try different rackets, at least two different days for each one (people usually hit great with a racket they are using for the first time). Avoid any tendency to buy a racket because a particular pro uses it. Or because you like its design or color. Take everything into consideration about the racket's playing characteristics and match them to your game.

A TANGLED WEB OF STRINGS

Just as you would fit an expensive guitar with quality strings, a prized tennis racket deserves the same. But it isn't necessary to pay the cost for gut strings (made from, yes, the intestines of animals). While gut will deliver lively shots, synthetics are quite comparable. Nylon is the most common material, but other synthetics are also used. String construction may be of solid cores with outer wraps (for crisp shot response), multiple filament cores with outer wraps (for better cushioning), textured outer wraps (to aid spin), or hybrids for overall performance.

The higher a string's gauge, the thinner it is. Thinner strings (16- or 17-gauge) are livelier, while thicker strings (15- or 15L-gauge) are more durable. Overall, 16-gauge is a sensible medium.

The effect of varying string tension is rather confusing. Laboratory tests generally indicate that a lower tension (within reason) will produce a higher ball velocity, because looser strings are more deflected by ball impact and will respond with a trampoline effect as the energy stored by the strings is returned to the ball as its flung into rebound. Higher string tension causes the ball to be more flattened out during impact, in turn increasing the imbedding of the ball into the strings with a greater contact area, and consequently giving the ball more control. Relatedly, the trampoline effect of loose strings holds the ball on the racket face longer, thus on off-center hits the racket has more time to rotate and send the ball off course.

However, it's not all that conclusive, for it seems that each racket has vibration and power qualities that are specific to its design. Manufacturers have performed tests on their products, and have recommended tension ranges for each racket for optimal performance. Stringing a racket outside these ranges will not match the tension with the mechanics of the racket.

IF THE SHOE FITS

When you slam the 26 bones of each foot into the court for three sets your shoes need to provide cushioning and durability. The force of foot impact on the court is most often absorbed by the heel, therefore any shoe you buy needs to fit snug on your heel to keep your foot from slithering around inside the shoe and to distribute the shock more evenly.

If you are a serve and volley player the shoe should also have a firm toe cap to absorb the forward stopping and starting. If you are a baseline player, the sidewalls must be substantial, or perhaps a hi-top shoe should be worn. If you play on clay there are shoes designed to allow a slide, but they will not be as adequate for quick changes of direction on hard-surface courts.

Test the shoe in the store for flexibility and firmness at the right places. Twist it, bend it, flex it. Avoid any extremes, especially in midfoot flexibility — neither a too stiff shoe or one that is too pliable. Put your best foot (feet?) forward with shoes that give stability, comfort, and resilience.

Appendix A

Aerobic Conditioning for Tennis

An hour or more of tennis — it isn't the most physically brutal thing you can do to yourself. But to play consistently excellent tennis requires both a well-rehearsed stroke repertoire and a ready state of physical preparedness. This is increasingly true as you move up the skill ladder, where rallies become longer and points more intensively contested. So you'll need reserves of (1) **strength**, to hit the ball hard and to get from here to there in a hurry, (2) **endurance**, to go full-out from beginning to the end of a match, and (3) **flexibility**, to reach high and bend low and swing unrestricted through a full range of motion.

STRENGTH

Tennis does not make uncompromising demands for brute strength. But being responsively strong will help you get quickly from one side of the court to the other, or to more effectively block a crushing serve, or to put more drive into your groundstrokes. Furthermore, it will improve the probability of staying injury-free.

You need **explosive power** — the ability to contract muscles quickly. Consequently, disciplined exercises should concentrate on weight **training** instead of weight **lifting**. Weight training is using lighter weights and more repetition of movement than weight lifting. The product is muscles that are alert and responsive for the quick-trigger action of a tennis match.

Give special attention to the muscles on the front of the thighs (the quadriceps) and the back of the thighs (hamstrings); the upper back and shoulder (trapezius and deltoids); and the back of the upper arm (triceps). Remember that any workout with weights should be preceded by a warm-up, including stretching, and should take the muscles through a full range of motion without pushing to the point of strain.

ENDURANCE

To prepare for long, intense matches, you need some off-court exercises that will elevate your heart rate to at least 120 beats a minute and keep it there for 20 or 30 minutes, three times a week minimum. Walking won't do it. Nor will a leisurely bike ride. But an energetic jog will — or anything else that has you perspiring freely after ten minutes.

That will help you maintain your peak performance as a match wears on. But the game-by-game demands are stop-and-go. So the training program should also include lots of sprint-type bursts of energy.

You can easily include these in a jogging regimen. Jog for a given distance, then sprint for ten full strides, then jog again, then sprint ten strides, and so on. Or come to a sudden stop and run backwards a short distance. Or sideways. Or twist your upper body as you run like you were hitting groundstrokes. In these actions you'll be imitating the moves of a tennis match, besides adding variety to the jogging.

FLEXIBILITY

When your muscles are supple and your joints flexible, you'll be better able to spring into a flat-out run for chasing down a wide ball. And you'll more easily crank the racket into the arched position for a topspin serve. And you'll be more responsive to get your racket on every ball at the net.

Moreover, these moments of sudden exertion are when muscle pulls occur. But you can reduce the risk by a conscientious program of stretching. And stretching after a match, when your muscles are warm and limber and can be extended fully, will help eliminate soreness and stiffness.

Remember:
- Do only static stretching. No bouncing! Curiously, bouncing actually works **against** the development of flexibility, because a muscle that is quickly stretched will react by contracting, thus resisting the stretch and increasing the chances of being torn during the exercise. So stretch **slowly**. And hold the end position for a few seconds.
- Don't push to pain. If it hurts, stop. Pain is your body's way of telling you to go easy. Don't force the stretching, and what was uncomfortable today will be an easy position to achieve next week.

CIRCUIT TRAINING

Circuit training involves a series of stations, spread out over a jogging course, each

Appendix A: Aerobic Conditioning for Tennis

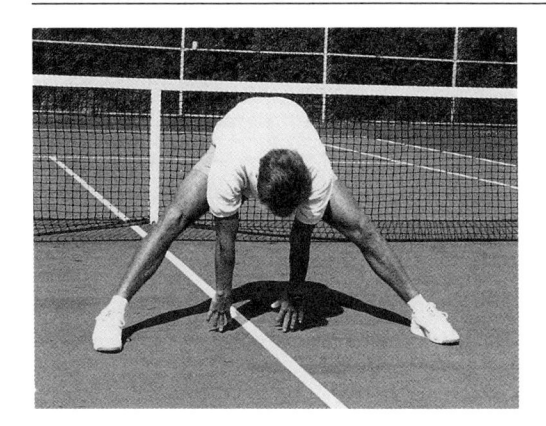

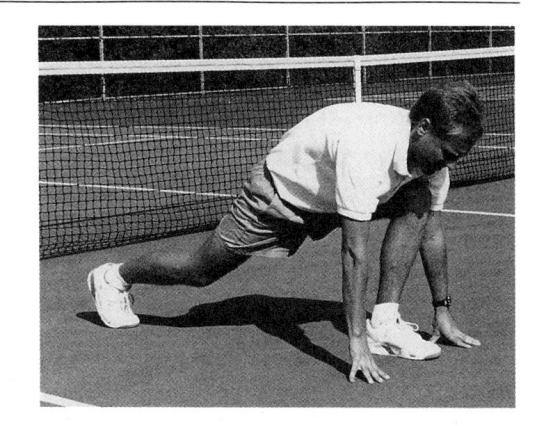

Before a match, after a short warm-up, stretch your muscles out, for three reasons: (1) it will reduce the risk of a muscle pull, (2) it helps to elevate the temperature of your muscles, and (3) it gets your muscles into a responsive state, more prepared for the job you have for them.

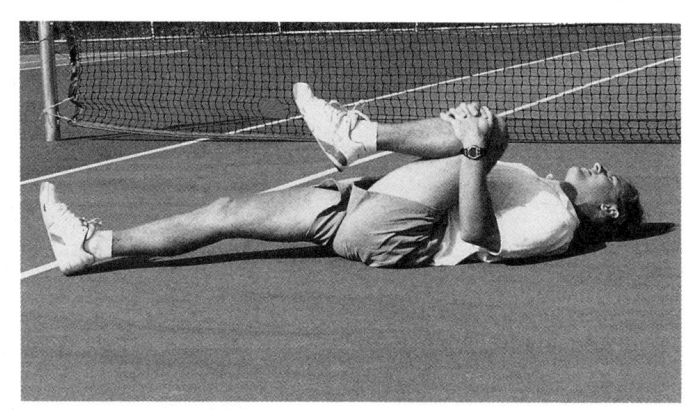

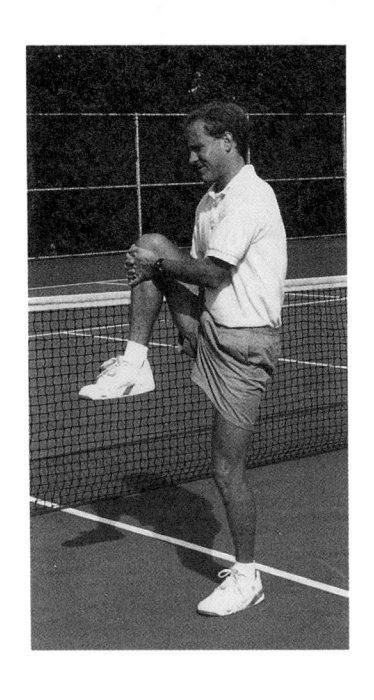

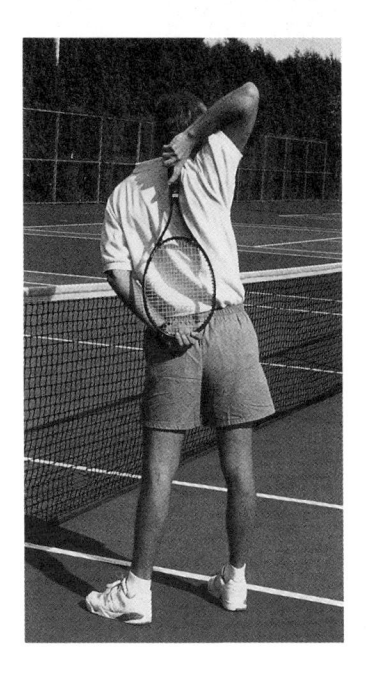

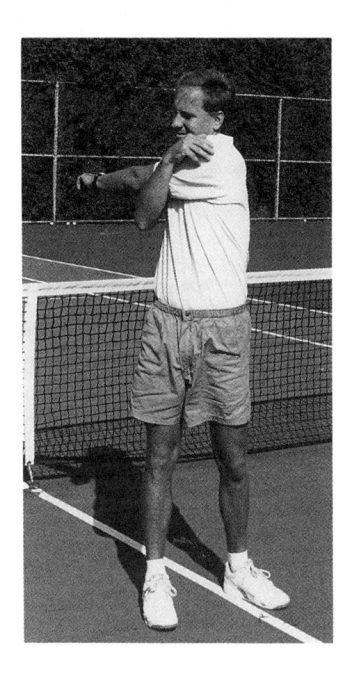

station having a specific exercise routine. As you come to each station you perform the given exercise, then walk, jog, or run to the next station where another exercise will be performed. The objective is to complete the circuit in as short a time as possible, and/or to increase the number or repetitions at each station whenever the course is run.

Circuit training is terrific conditioning for tennis. It fosters the kind of physical preparation that is needed for the game. And the circuit is individualized, because you set your own pace and number of repetitions. Best of all, if you do not have an already designed course available, you can easily create your own circuit, without any need of equipment. Just try to add a combination of strength, endurance, and flexibility exercises in the plan. Start with a warm-up, then some stretching, and jog for a distance in-between each of the exercises illustrated below and on the next page, as examples.

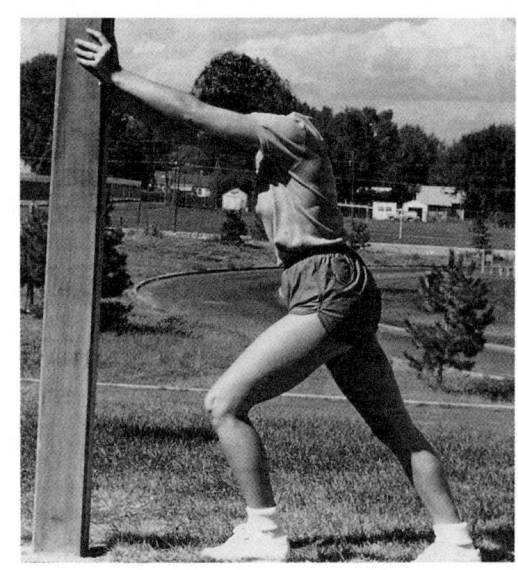

Start by doing some stretching.

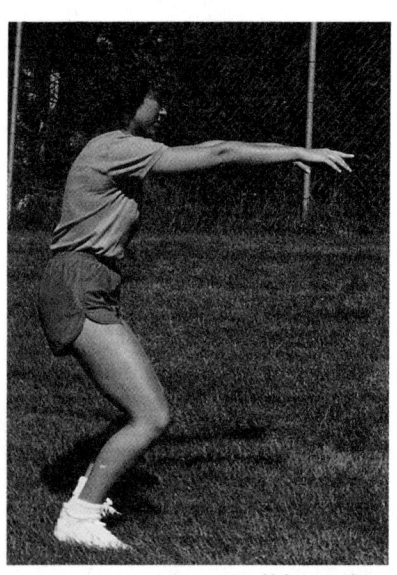

Half-knee dips.

Bent-knee situps.

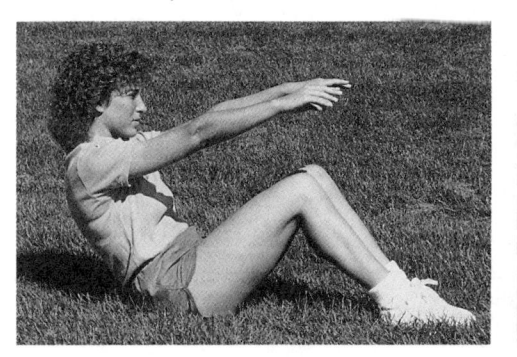

Push up off ground, clap hands.

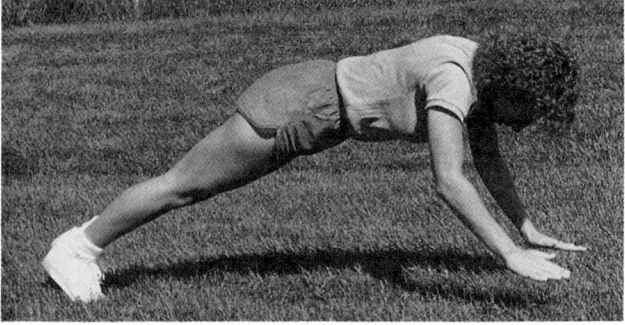

Appendix A: Aerobic Conditioning for Tennis 143

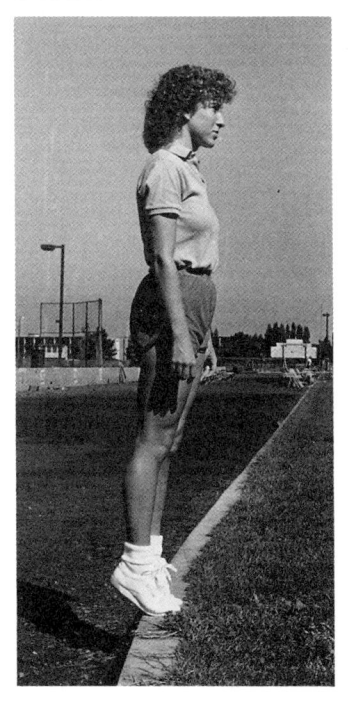

Heel raises.

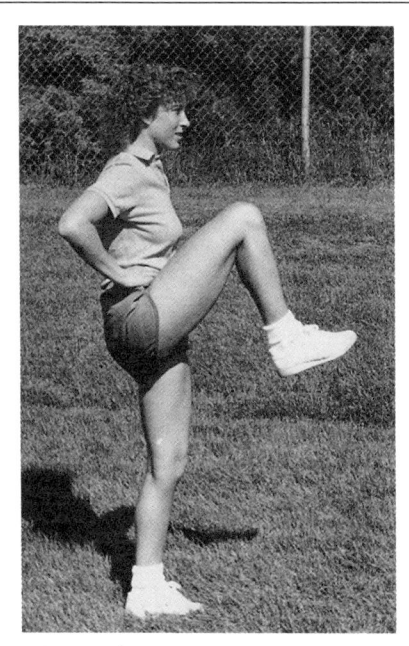

Knee raises.

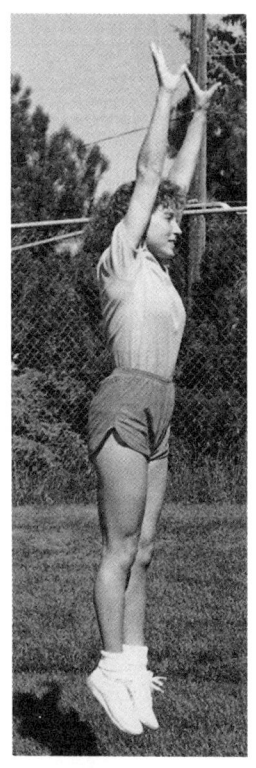

Jump and reach.

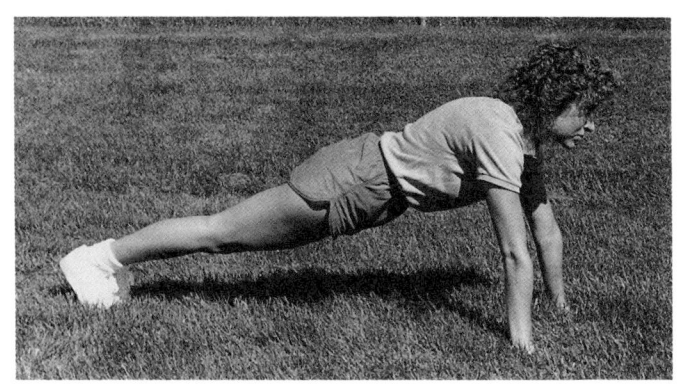

Pushups.

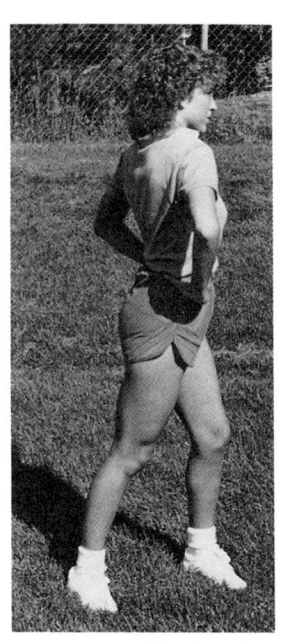

Trunk twists.

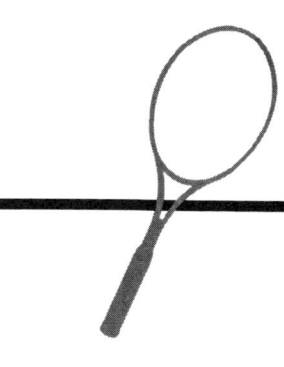

Appendix B

History
Game

Ma... nused corner of the grounds. But the game
in Be... ound little favor with club members.
Januar... Women saw it as unladylike, and men con-
diers ...ersely thought it too genteel (and it was
over ...asy to snub a game where "love" was part of
quick ...he scoring).
becan
equip   Despite this early rejection of tennis,
her h within a few years it was included as an
activity at nearly every major cricket club in
toms officials debated for a week over what the east, and soon its popularity would over-
duty should be levied on the paraphernalia, step its aristocratic boundaries to become a
then allowed it to enter tax free, and there- sport of the masses. It continued to grow,
upon tennis had its first entry into the slowly and steadily, then experienced a mani-
United States. fold increase in participants during the
1960s and 1970s to where today there are 20
As a member of the Staten Island Cricket million Americans who play tennis on a reg-
and Baseball Club, Miss Outerbridge ular basis.
received permission to lay out a court on an

The earliest origins of the game are much more obscure. A study of ancient cultures reveals that a game of batting a ball over an obstacle was played 2,000 years ago in Greece, perhaps also during the Roman Empire, and in the Orient, where the first rackets may have been used.

Despite the obscurity of the ancient origins of tennis, there is no doubt that a tennis-like game was played in the parks and chateaus of thirteenth-century France. Called by the name of jeu de paume (literally, game of the hand), it was first a barehanded game of hitting a stuffed cloth bag over a rope. Rackets were not used until the late fifteenth or early sixteenth century. As enthusiasm for the activity spread, larger towns, not having ample outdoor space, began building indoor courts in anything from cowsheds to monasteries. (In fact, monks were some of the earliest players.)

Jeu de paume met with some unfavorable reactions in its early times, even to the point of being outlawed in a few areas, but the general popularity of the game continued to climb. The growing acceptance did not wane even though King Louis X died in 1316, allegedly from a chill caught while playing a tennis match. Most of the fourteenth-century Kings took up the sport, and the masses now found major recreation in it. And, by the close of the fourteenth century the game was well established in Holland and in England, where the writings of Chaucer indicate that it was called by its present name, tennis, probably a derivation of the French word "tenez," which was originally a call made by the server before putting the ball into play.

In France, as the game became a more prominent social enterprise, monetary wagers on tennis matches soon became commonplace. Such practice encouraged professionalism, and by the beginning of the fifteenth century there were 1,400 professional players in France, even though the first written rules did not appear until 1599. In spite of the prevalence of gambling, tennis reached a peak of popularity in both England and France during the sixteenth and seventeenth centuries; Paris alone having built 1,800 courts. But the scandalous exchange of money almost obliterated the sport in the middle of the eighteenth century, and when the dust had settled from the French Revolution there was only one court remaining in use in Paris.

Civil war also depressed the playing of tennis in England, although the upper classes continued in their zeal for the sport. Then, in 1873, British Army Major Walter C. Wingfield introduced his guests at a garden party to a new outdoor game, played on an hourglass court, but with many of the characteristics of present-day tennis. Major Wingfield referred to the activity as "sphairistike," claiming it was the same game the ancient Greeks had played (sphairistike in Greek connotates "to play"). The English populace was rapidly caught up with this new version of the game, and soon there were courts throughout the country. Four years later, in 1877, the court was changed to its present rectangular shape, and a new code of rules was established that has remained remarkably the same in context to those of today. Also in 1877, the world's first major tennis championships were held at Wimbledon, a southwest suburb of London, which has continued as the site of one of the four "Grand Slam" tournaments in the world (along with the championships of France, Australia, and the United States).

There was an army officer at Major Wingfield's party in 1873 who took the game with him to Bermuda as a pastime for the British garrison stationed there. Enter Mary Outerbridge.

Appendix C

The National Tennis Rating Program

The National Tennis Association has developed a self-rating scale as a method of classifying skill levels for more compatible matches, group lessons, league play, tournaments, and other programs. For example, a tournament may be listed as a 3.5 tournament and it is expected that, to insure equitable competition, only players of that level will enter.

The National Tennis Rating Program: General Characteristics of Various Playing Levels

1.0 This player is just starting to play tennis.

1.5 This player has limited experience and is still working primarily on getting the ball into play.

2.0 This player needs on-court experience. This player has obvious stroke weaknesses but is familiar with basic positions for singles and doubles play.

2.5 This player is learning to judge where the ball is going although court coverage is weak. This player can sustain a rally of slow pace with other players of the same ability.

3.0 This player is consistent when hitting medium paced shots, but is not comfortable with all strokes and lacks control when trying for directional intent, depth, or power.

3.5 This player has achieved improved stroke dependability and direction on moderate shots, but still lacks depth and variety. This player is starting to exhibit more aggressive net play, has improved court coverage, and is developing teamwork in doubles.

4.0 This player has dependable strokes, including directional intent and depth on both forehand and backhand sides on moderate shots, plus the ability to use lobs, overheads, approach shots and volleys with some success. This player occasionally forces errors when serving and teamwork in doubles is evident.

4.5 This player has begun to master the use of power and spins and is beginning to handle pace, has sound footwork, can control depth of shots, and is beginning to vary tactics according to opponents. This player can hit first serves with power and accuracy and place the second serve and is able to rush net successfully. Aggressive net play is common in doubles.

5.0 This player has good shot anticipation and frequently has an outstanding shot or attribute around which a game may be structured. This player can regularly hit winners or force errors off of short balls and can put away volleys, can successfully execute lobs, drop shots, half volleys and overhead smashes and has good depth and spin on most second serves.

5.5 This player has developed power and or consistency as a major weapon. This player can vary strategies and styles of play in a competitive situation and hits dependable shots in a stress situation.

6.0 to 7.0 These players will generally not need NTRP ratings. Rankings or past rankings will speak for themselves. The 6.0 player typically has had intensive training for national tournament competition at the junior level and collegiate levels and has obtained a sectional and/or national ranking. The 6.5 player has a reasonable chance of succeeding at the 7.0 level and has extensive satellite tournament experience. The 7.0 is a world class player who is committed to tournament competition on the international level and whose major source of income is tournament prize winnings.

Appendix D

A Self-Appraisal Checklist of Skill

What follows here is a series of reminders about the essentials of each aspect of tennis. The list does not include everything that is important, but rather some of the most important factors.

Use the list to build your own mental cue system for performance. Keep the cues brief, so that on the court you can use a small package of information to remind your body of the things it ought to be doing.

Take the list along to the court. Check the appropriate box for each item on the list, or have someone else evaluate your performance. Use the checklist as a reference, noting those parts of your game which need more practice time.

PERFORMANCE CUES

	Usually performed	Sometimes performed	Rarely performed
For all strokes:			
1. Stay relaxed, yet alive, limber, alert, and responsive.			
2. Hit as if the racket is a part of you — an extension of your arm.			
3. Make every stroke fluid, free-flowing, rhythmical.			
4. Hit the ball with your entire body, not just your arm.			
5. Keep the racket alive — active through contact. Emphasize the follow-through.			
6. Play dynamic, lively, spontaneous tennis.			
7. Enjoy the sensory stimulus of the game itself.			
For the groundstrokes:			
1. Stay athletic, lively on your toes, cat-like on the court.			
2. Keep the grip loose to start — firm to hit.			
3. Coil and uncoil — everything back to wind up, forward to hit.			
4. Have your weight going toward the target at contact.			
5. Hit low-to-high for topspin, with a firm wrist at contact.			
6. Fling the racket into the ball for topspin, with good acceleration at contact.			
7. Hit high to low for backspin, with a firm wrist at contact.			

Appendix D: A Self-Appraisal Checklist of Skill

	Usually performed	Sometimes performed	Rarely performed
For the Serve			
1. Close the stance; take a Continental grip.			
2. Keep a loose, supple arm.			
3. Spiral your whole body into the backswing, racket head down.			
4. Start slow, but explode into the ball, with a whip-like action.			
5. Hit both serves with the same intensity; change only the direction of the swing.			
For the return of serve:			
1. Prime yourself to move forward.			
2. Be lively on your feet; ready to move quickly.			
3. The harder the serve, the more the swing should be compact and firm.			
4. Be a scrambler. Go to the ball. Don't retreat. Do anything to get the ball back.			
When playing the forecourt:			
1. Go to the net only on a short ball or behind your own strong shot.			
2. Hit the approach shot deep.			
3. As your opponent is about to hit, come to a split-step pause.			

	Usually performed	Sometimes performed	Rarely performed
4. Keep the volley stroke firm, compact.			
5. For an overhead, get into position early, behind the ball.			
6. Hit the smash with flair, but only as hard as you can control.			
7. Defend the net aggressively, like a goalkeeper defending the goal.			
When hitting lobs:			
1. Hit the lob as an offensive weapon whenever you can.			
2. Hit defensive lobs with plenty of height.			
3. Keep a firm wrist for all lobs except topspin, which needs wrist.			
4. Bring the racket into the ball on the same plane as the intended loft of the shot.			
In pressure situations:			
1. When hitting on the run, shorten the backswing, give the arm whip, provide margin of safety for placement.			
2. Hit half-volleys with firm wrist; racket parallel to court, push the ball back deep.			
3. Hit a high backhand like a volley; firm grasp, push racket forward.			
4. When retreating from the net to catch up to a lob, hit a lob in return.			

	Usually performed	Sometimes performed	Rarely performed
On touch shots:			
1. Slacken the grip for drop shots. Bunt the ball over the net.			
2. Use drop shots, or dink the ball, only when you know that you can end the point with the shot.			
As strategy for singles:			
1. Keep the ball deep, and up the middle, especially against a strong groundstroke player.			
2. Use angled shots when you're shallow and/or off to one side.			
3. Beat a slugger with changes of pace, and lots of off-speed shots.			
4. Go to the forecourt often: finish the point early; hit the ball where your opponent isn't.			
5. Make things happen. Try to win points rather than trying to avoid losing them.			
6. Get the first serve in at least half the time; slow its pace if necessary.			
7. Hit second serves to the weaker side of the receiver.			
8. Do what you do best, and play it against what your opponent does worst.			
As strategy for doubles:			
1. Go to the net at every opportunity.			

	Usually performed	Sometimes performed	Rarely performed
2. Sacrifice pace for placement.			
3. Get first serves in more often. Send them to receiver's weaker side.			
4. When at the net, as partner of server or receiver, take every ball you can get.			
5. Return serves past net player, low in front of server.			
6. Lob more often, and exploit the middle.			
As states of mind:			
1. Self-talk optimism into your mind; believe in your own ability.			
2. Maintain a state of calm, even during stressful points of a match.			
3. Focus on each point, as if it were the last of the match.			
4. Believe that every serve will go in. See the ball good before hitting it.			
5. Do not let a poor shot affect your performance on the next shot.			
6. Keep an upbeat attitude, and competitive spirit, for the entire match.			
7. Use visualization, both off the court and during breaks in a match.			

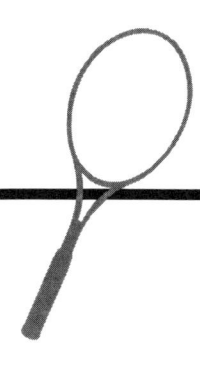

Appendix E

The Rules of Tennis

The official rules that govern tennis are a product of the International Tennis Federation, of which the United States Tennis Association (USTA) is a member. They are presented in complete form at the end of this chapter. However, there is a certain "spirit" of the rules and codes of conduct which are first discussed.

Implied Integrity

No tradition in tennis is older than that of integrity among players. This integrity starts through having a complete knowledge of the rules and the ethical codes that oblige every player to do nothing which detracts from the game itself, or from an opponent's concentration on their own play. This includes giving an opponent the benefit of doubt on line calls, avoiding foot faults during serving, never intentionally distracting an opponent, never stalling, and always conducting oneself in a fashion that makes the game enjoyable for everyone. In this way, honest players will have the same approach to all situations, and the competitive ideals of tennis will remain high.

Line Calls

A dozen or more times in every set a ball lands so near a line that it's difficult to tell, accurately, if it was in or out. Here are some hypothetical situations regarding that occurrence.

1. During a rally you keep a ball in play that you realize was out. Can you make a delayed call of "out" and claim the point?

● No. Any call of "out" must be made as soon as possible. Otherwise, a player could watch their return go out-of-bounds and then decide to make the "out" call on the opponent's previous placement.

2. Suppose your opponent's first serve and your return of that serve happen so fast that you have sent the ball back over the net before you have concluded in your mind that the ball was actually out.

● The same principle applies: the ball must be called out right away. However, there is some allowance in this instance, because it is understood that the receiver is concentrating first on returning the ball, second on making the call. But in no case can the call be made after the ball has either been sent back into the opposing court or has been hit out-of-bounds.

3. What if your opponent hits a point-ending placement that you are not sure was in or out — must you still make an immediate call?

● In this case, time permits you to have a "second look" at the placement, sometimes even finding a mark left by the ball, before making the call.

4. Can you ask for a replay of a point where you are unable to make a sure call?

● Absolutely not! The rules do not allow it. Whenever there is doubt, that doubt must be resolved in favor of your opponent; therefore, unless you clearly saw the ball as out, it must be considered to have been good.

5. Can you ask your opponent to make the call on a ball you did not clearly see?

● Yes, but only when you believe that your opponent was in a better position to see the ball than you were. Usually this happens when you are looking **across** a line and your opponent is looking **down** the line at the placement. The player looking down the line is more likely to have accurately seen the ball than a player looking across a line.

6. Should you enlist the aid of a spectator to help make a line call?

● Never. It is discourteous to your opponent, an avoidance of your responsibility, and does not guarantee accuracy or impartiality on the part of the spectator.

7. Suppose you hit a point-ending placement that you clearly saw as out and your opponent calls good. Should you correct the call, and as a result lose the point?

● Yes; even if your opponent does not ask you to make the call.

8. Suppose you hit a serve you see as out, but your opponent nevertheless returns the ball without making an "out" call. Could you ask for a replay on the basis that the

return was unexpected and caught you unprepared for continuance of play?

- It must be assumed that the receiver made the return in good faith, thinking the serve to be good; therefore, play must continue, with no allowance for a replay. However, there is a general guideline that the server (or the server's partner in doubles) should volunteer a call on a **second** serve that is clearly seen as out, since this call terminates the point.

One rather awkward situation is when a player sees a ball which is apparently going out and then catches the ball before it lands. The rules clearly state that the player automatically loses the point, since the ball is alive as long as it's in the air and therefore cannot be touched by a player. However, sometimes a player will catch a ball before it bounces simply to keep it from rebounding over a fence or into a neighboring court; thus some discretion must be used in the exact letter of this rule. Making a call against an opponent who caught a ball unquestionably going out-of-bounds, though lawfully correct, may be ethically unsound when that player was merely trying to conserve time by not having to collect the errant ball after its bounce.

The Let

Sometimes an event occurs which prevents a player from having full concentration on the point being played. Such is the case when, for example, a player is distracted by a ball coming from another court, or by players walking around or behind the court. This distraction allows the hindered player to legally call a let, with the privilege of replaying the point. However, the let must be called **right away.** This prevents any player from having a "two chance" option whereby that player was, for instance, hindered by a ball from another court but continues to play the point and, having hit the ball out, then tries to exercise the let. Furthermore, a let cannot be called when there was a hindrance but the player had absolutely no chance of retrieving a good placement from their opponent.

Note that a replayed point begins with the server being granted the normal two attempts. In effect, this means that if the server was hindered or otherwise interrupted during or before the **second** serve attempt, the rules allow for the server to have **both** attempts over again. However, the concept of an "inordinate delay" should be applied in this circumstance. That is, unless there is an inordinate amount of time between serves caused by that hindrance, a let should not be allowed, and the server must carry on with the second attempt. But when the server is forced, by some reason not of their doing, to wait an unreasonable length of time to hit the second attempt, the **receiver** should acknowledge that fact and "grant" the server the privilege to start again with the first serve. This is a prime example of the importance for all players to know the rules so that the receiver in this case not only understands what should be done, but also observes the courtesy of recognizing the event which allows the server to have both attempts.

That Bothersome Foot Fault

Everybody does it now and then, usually unknowingly. But what do you do if your opponent commits repeated and blatant foot faults?

The rules have no provision about what to do, but a USTA interpretation of the foot fault authorizes the receiver to first inform the server of the violation and then, if it continues, to make a call. However, the call should be made only when the receiver is absolutely certain of the violation.

It's irritating. When you are receiving, you do not want to be bothered with having to give some attention to watching for a foot fault; therefore, the only ones that you are likely to notice are the flagrant violations. But even the slightest encroachment on the line is still a foot fault, and thus compliance with this rule is very much a function of each player's sense of honor.

Other Considerations

Following are some additional matters which, when understood by all players, will make for a better and more enjoyable match.

1. Whenever a player realizes that they have committed a violation, that player should make the call immediately. This includes such things as hitting the ball after two bounces, touching the net, or hitting the ball before it has crossed over the net.
2. If a player calls a ball out, then realizes that it was good, a correction should be made.
3. The server should announce the score of the set prior to the first serve of a new game, and the score of the game prior to serving each point. Always, the server's score is announced first, the receiver's second.
4. If there is disagreement among the players as to the score and it cannot be resolved, the score shall revert back to the last score on which there was agreement, or it should be settled by the spin of a racket.
5. Although a receiver may change their position on the court as the server prepares to hit or begins the motion, this must not be done in a deliberate attempt to disrupt the server.
6. Sometimes a server will, having missed a first attempt, hit the second serve before the receiver has had ample time to assume a ready position. While this is a violation on the part of the server, the receiver must also recognize that even when being victimized by such a "quick serve," if any overt attempt is made to return the ball, the receiver forfeits the right to ask for a replay of the second serve.
7. Stalling in an attempt to unnerve an opponent is not permitted.
8. Intentionally returning serves that are out in an effort to upset an opponent is not to be tolerated.
9. During the warm-up prior to the start of a match, it is courtesy to keep the ball within easy reach of the opponent and to refrain from returning the ball when the opponent is practicing serves.
10. All practice serves should be taken during the warm-up instead of allowing the second server of the match to practice serves prior to their first turn, after the first game has been completed.

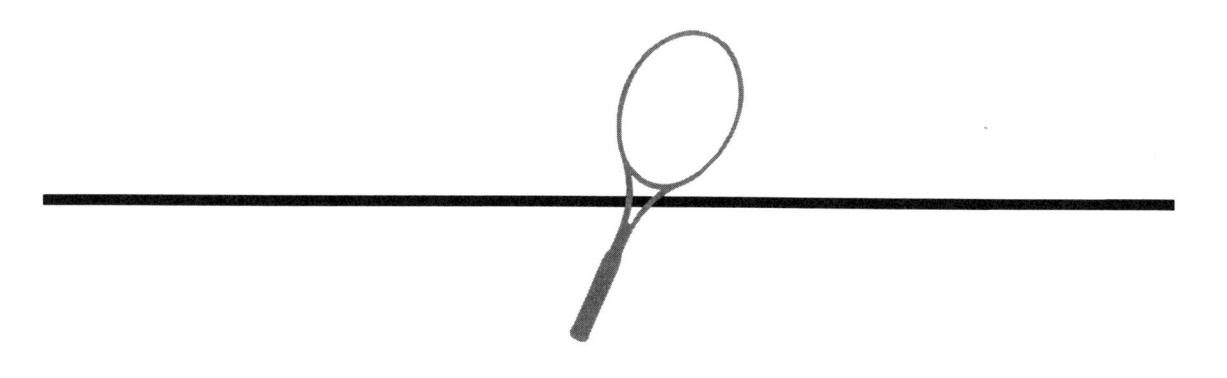

INDEX

Note: page numbers in italics refer to photographs and illustrations.

acceleration, of racket, 12, 31
acting like a winner, 123
ad court, 107-108, *116*
advantage court. See court
aerobic conditioning, 139-143
aerobic workout, 130-134
All-Court Scramble, *133*
alertness, 3
alley, 112
angles, use of, 94-95, *95*
anticipation, of failure, 123
"anything goes" shot. See shots
approach, line of, *109*
approach shots. See shots.
arching, of back, 37
arm, propelling racket, 84, 90
art, of tennis, 10
attention
　on ball, 2
　on what is relevant to performance, 121
attitude, mental, 1
Australian formation, 116, *116, 117*

backhand, 15, *15*, 31, 47, 72
　double-jointed, 83
　high, *85,* 85-86
　one-handed, 24
　smash, 86, *86*
　topspin, 24, *24*

backhand (continued)
　two-handed, 15, *16*, 24
backpedaling, 51, 68
backspin. See spin
backswing, 15, *15*, 22-23, 26, 36, 60, *63*, 68, 122
　delaying of, 83-84
balance, 19
ball
　flying too far, 29
　hitting at top of bounce, 60
　hit too long, 71
　into net, 29, 71
　late ball contact, 66
　problem solving for lobs, 81
　short, 94
　trying to hit too hard, 94
　wide, *66*, 94
　overpowering racket, 26
baseline, *60*, 94, 95
　players, 97
bent-knee situps, *142*
biofeedback, 1
blocking, of ball, 67
body language, 122
body position, *27*
"bounce," 3
"bounce step," 10, *58*

centering, on yourself, 121

161

charging the net, 55
Checklist of Skills, Self-Appraisal, 151-156
choreography, for overhead, 68
circuit training, 140-142, *142*
closing out opponent, 123-124
coil, 4, *4*, 72
competitive instinct, loss of, 123-124
confidence, competitive, 93
consistency, 10
constructive thought, 120
Continental grip, 34, 35, *35*, 71-72
control, of yourself, 122
Coriolis Effect, 101
Corner Rally, *131*
court
   advantage, 61
   deuce, 61
court surfaces, effects of, 104-105
creativity, importance of, 90
cross-over step, *66*
cutting, off of ball, 83

deep returns, 55
defensive
   position and lobs, 79
   tennis, 129
depth, 11, 97, 103
deuce court. See court
dimension, to shots, 129
double-helix pattern, 37
doubles play
   mixed, 117
   server's starting position in, *109*
   See also match play
drilling the ball, 61, *64*
drills
   practice, 72
   volley, 72
drop shots. See shots
drop volley. See volley

elbow, hitting, 75
emergency situations, responding to, 90
emotions, how they affect play, 119
empty space, covering in doubles play, 115
endurance, 139, 140
energy, for the hit, 37
energy, positive, 121
enjoyment, of game, 2
equipment, 120, 135-138
evaluation, of opponent, 121

exploitation, of middle, 112-113
eye on the ball, 8, *8*, 68, *68*, 81

fakery, 108-110
feet, of server, 51
finesse, use of, 89, 107
finish, 37
finishing instinct, 61
flexibility, 139, 140, *141*
floating, through strokes, 10
flow, of game, *1*
fluidity, of strokes, 2
focus, on ball. See eye on ball
follow-through, 7, 8, *14*, *27*, 30, 37, *43*, 60, 75, *76*
foot faults, 160
footwork, 10
forced wide, 62
force-vector advantage, 101
forecourt
   control of, 59-72
   use of, 97-98
forehand, *4*, 23, *27*, 31, 91
   running, 83
forward-at-contact impulse, 5
forward impact, 5, *6*, *7*
forward, moving, 112
Four-Ball Rally, 130
frames, racket, 135-136
France, 146

"Grand Slam" tournaments, 147
graphite, 135
Greeks, 146
grip, 11
   Continental. See Continental grip
   forehand. See forehand
   relaxing of, 90
groundstroke, 11-31, *74*, 98
   players, 95
   reminders, 18

half-knee dips, *142*
half-volley. See volley
hand shifting, 72
heel raises, *142*
history, of tennis, 145-147
Hit-and-advance, *131*
hitting
   down on the ball, 62
   free, 130

Index

hitting (continued)
  on the run, 83-84
  placement, 129
  purposeless, 128
  through ball, 7, *7*, 12, 37, 62
  too late, 56
honesty, with yourself, 120
human backboard, 97

impact, going forward at, 5
integrity, implied, 157

jump and reach, *142*

"kicker," 34
knee raises, *142*
knees, bending of, 8, 24, 37, 75, 85

lazy racket, 8, 128
left-handedness, 41, 101
let, 159
lights, effects of, 104
line calls, 157-158
lobs, 68-70, *68, 70*
  backhand, *76*
  backspin, 76, *79*
  cross-court, 79
  deep, return of, 86-89, *87*
  defensive, 73, 75, *77*
  hitting point-winning, 73-82
  influence of, in doubles play, 113, *113, 114*
  in match play, 79-80
  offensive, 73, *74,* 75, 79, *80,* 98, *114*
  problem solving, 81
  reminders, 80
  spin for, 75-76, *78*
  topspin, 75-76, *78*
Louis X, King, 146
lunging, for wide ball, 66

Machine-Gun Volleys, *132*
making things happen, 123
margin, of safety, 84
match play
  and lobs, 79-80
  doubles, 107-117. See also strategy, laws for doubles play
  singles, 93-105. See also strategy, laws for singles play
mental practice, 125
mental toughness, 119-125
momentum
  linear, 12, 13, *13, 14, 16, 17,* 19, *24*

momentum (continued)
  rotary, 12, 13, *13, 14, 16,* 19, *24, 27*
muscle memory, 128

National Tennis Rating Program, 149-150
negative mistakes, 122
negative states of mind, 119
net play, 59-72
  at the net, 61-65
  how to approach net, 60-61, *61, 62*
  problem solving for, 66
  when to approach net, 59-60, *60*
net rushers, 98, *99*
neural pathways, 128
"no-man's land," 71
"nothing" ball, 96

offensive tennis, 128-129
open position, 13, 15
Outerbridge, Mary, 145, 147
overheads, 68-69, *68, 69, 88*
  lunging, 83

pace, 11, 56-57, 60, 65, 96, 100
Palmer, Arnold, 123
patience, 98-99, 107
percentage tennis, 105
pivot, whole-body, 4, *4*
placement, of shots, 11, 55-56, 57, 60, *64,* 67, 94-95, 100, 107
poaching, 108-110, *110, 111*
point-finishing instinct, 71
points, 61
position, in doubles, 107
positive tennis, 122-123
positive thinking, 2
power
  adding to topspin serves, 37-39
  hitters, 96-97, *96*
  lack of, 9
  sources of, 12
practice, realistic, 127-134
practice session, 129-130
problem solving, 9, 19, 29, 45, 56-57, 66, 71
push-ups, *142, 143*

racket
  acceleration, 12
  analyzing a, 136
  and topspin serves, 34
  buying a, 136-137

racket (continued)
  characteristics, 135-136
  chopping, 24
  design, 135
  face, tilting for lob, 68, *74*
  how it produces spin, 22, 25
  playability of, 136
  power, 37
  strings, 137
rain, effects of, 104
rapid fire, 129
readiness, physical, 120
ready position, 3, *3, 62*
rebound, 34
receive, practice, 130
receiver's partner, 112
recovery, 84
reflexes, and return of serve, 49, 57
rehearsal, of offense and defense, 128-129
relaxation, 2-3, 39, 93, 120, 124
reminders, 9, 19, 28, 44, 56, 65, 69, 80
response, sluggish, 9
return of serve, 49-58, 110-112
  down-the-line, 84
  getting ready, 50-51, *50*
  on the run, 83-84
  too long, 57
  when ball arrives, 51, *52, 53, 54*
  when ball is on the way, 50
  where to send ball, 55-56
  where to stand, 49-50, *50*
rhythm, 2-3
rotation, ball, 20-21, *20*
rules, of tennis, 157-160

scissors act, *111, 115*
self-talk, 124
sequence, of shots, 98-100, *100*
serve, 33-47
  attacking second, 104
  Australian formation, 116, *116, 117*
  directly at receiver, 102
  down-the-middle, 100
  far-corner, 102
  first, 39-41, 102
  flat, 34, 36, *36, 42-43*
  forceful, *54*
  getting first serve in, 102
  hard, 51
  into net, 45
  kick, 103

serve (continued)
  minimal ball rotation, 45
  not enough topspin, 45
  practice, 46, *46*, 130
  power, 45
  receiver's partner, 112
  return of, 49-58, 110-112, *111*
  second, 39-41, 46, *46*, 47, 58, 102-103, 104
  slice, 41, *42-43*, 58
  strategy in doubles, 108
  too long, 45
  topspin, 33-34, 37, *38*, 39, *40*
  where to hit, 102-104, *103*
  wide, *52, 53*
Serve and Volley, *132*
server, partner of in doubles, 108
setup time, 129-130
shoes, 137-138
short ball, 59
shots
  angled, 112
  "anything goes," 90
  approach, 60
  cross-court, 65, 94
  drop, 89, *89*, 99, 101
  erratic, 19
  extraordinary, 83-91
  flat passing, 28
  hitting in sequence, 98-100
  lifeless, 9
  path of, 60
  put-away, 97
  specialty, 130
  strong, 59
  tight, jerky, 9
  touch, 89-90
  wide, 83-84
shuffle-step, 68, *70*
sidespin, 41
side-to-side relationship, *113, 114*
singles matches. See match play
slice. See serve
sluggers, 96-97
spin, 20-29, 100
  advantage of, 20
  backspin, 20, 21, *21*, 25, *26*, 28, 97
  effects of, 20-22
  how the racket produces, 22
  topspin, 20, *20*, 21, 22-25, *23*, 29, 30, *30*
  underspin. See backspin above
  using different styles of, 90-91

spin (continued)
  using in match play, 25-28
split-step, *58*, 60, *61*, *62*, 72
squared-off-to-the-net position, 35
stance
  receiving, 50-51, *50*
  serving, 34-35, *35*
standing, for receiving a serve, 49-50, *50*
stepping
  at the ball, *14*
  into the ball, *14*
straight-ahead approach, *109*
strategy, laws of for doubles play
  cover the empty space, 115, *115*
  exploiting the middle, 112-113
  fakery, 108-110
  get a good start, 107-108
  lobs, 113, *114*
  moving forward, 112
  poaching, 108-110, *110*, *111*
  return of serve, 110-112, *111*
  receiver's partner, 112
  server's partner, 108
  serving strategy, 108
  use of Australian formation, 116, *116*, *117*
strategy, law of for singles play
  adapting to court surface, 104-105
  against a net rusher, 98, *99*
  beating a human backboard, 97
  beating a slugger, 96-97
  beating a strong groundstroke player, 95, *96*
  beating the elements, 104
  getting first serve in, 102
  hitting shots in sequence, 98-100
  keep ball deep, 94
  keep ball in play, 93-94
  knowing when to use angles, 94-95, *95*
  left-handers, 101
  making things happen, 100-101
  playing percentage tennis, 105
  playing within your ability, 101
  use of forecourt, 97-98
  where to hit serve, 102-103, *103*
stress, before a match, 119-120
stretching, static, 140, *141*
strings, racket, 137
stroke
  for half-volley, *84*
  no strength to, 67
  preparation, 120
  volley, 65, 69

stutter-steps, 60, 83, 104
sun, effects of, 104
"sweet spot," 136
swing
  flattened arc, 15-17, *17*
  static-arm, *17*
  wraparound, 19

"T," 89
technique, keeping it within your ability, 101
Three-Shot Sequence, *134*
timeliness, 120
timing, 2-3
topspin. See spin
topspin motion, *88*, 89
toss, 36, *36*, *38*, *40*, 41, 57-58
"touch" shots, 89-90
trajectories, 90
trunk twists, *143*
two-step maneuver, *66*

uncoil, 4, *38*, 46
underspin. See spin
"up-and-back," *133*
  philosophy, 99

velocity, of swing, 12, 100
versatility, in strokes, 90
volley, 61, 62, *63*, 65
  down-the-line, 65
  drive, 61, *64*, 71
  drop, 90, *90*
  half, 83, *84*, 84-85

warm-up, pre-match, 120-121
weather, effects of, 104
weight training, 139-140
weight transfer, 12, 24
  improper, 9
Wimbledon, 146-147
wind, effects of, 104
windup, 12, 36-37, *38*, 68, *68*
Wingfield, Walter C., 146

wrist, 30, *30*, 34, 39, *65*, *70*, *74*, 90
wrong-footing an opponent, 75, 97